MW00979477

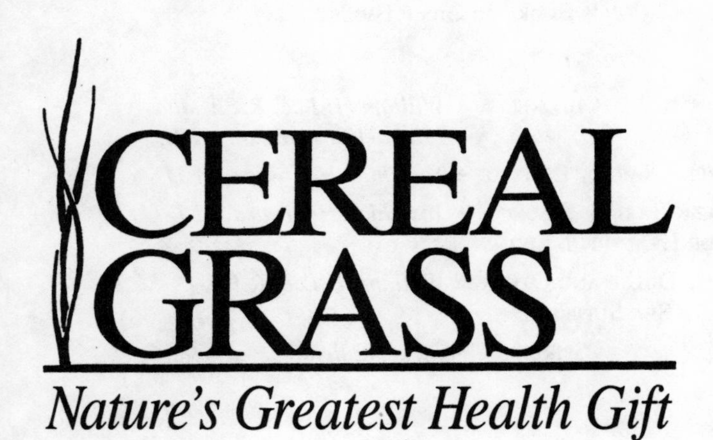
CEREAL
GRASS
Nature's Greatest Health Gift

Keats Books on Green Foods

CHLORELLA • *William H. Lee, R.Ph. and Michael Rosenbaum, M.D.*

GREEN BARLEY ESSENCE • *Yoshihide Hagiwara, M.D.*

GREEN BARLEY ESSENCE: RECIPES FOR HEALTHFUL LIVING • *Yoshihide Hagiwara, M.D.*

KELP, DULSE AND OTHER SEA SUPPLEMENTS • *William H. Lee, R.Ph.*

SPIRULINA • *Jack Challem*

CEREAL GRASS

Nature's Greatest Health Gift

Edited by
RONALD L. SEIBOLD, M.S.

KEATS PUBLISHING, INC. *New Canaan, Connecticut*

***Cereal Grass: Nature's Greatest Health Gift* is not intended as medical advice. Its intent is solely informational and educational. Please consult a health professional should the need for one be indicated.**

CEREAL GRASS: NATURE'S GREATEST HEALTH GIFT

Originally published by the Wilderness Community Education Foundation, Lawrence, Kansas under the title: *Cereal Grass: What's in It for You!*

Published by arrangement with the author

Cover design by Mark Schraad and Michael Stromberg

Back cover photo by Dwight Hilpman. Photo on page 100 by Margaret Moritz; all other photos by Ronald L. Seibold.

Library of Congress Cataloging-in-Publication Data

Cereal grass : nature's greatest health gift / edited by Ronald L. Seibold.
p. cm.
Reprint. Originally pub.: Lawrence, Kan. : Wilderness Community Education Foundation, 1990.
Includes bibliographical references and index.
ISBN 0-87983-631-8 ; $9.95
1. Cereal grasses in human nutrition. 2. Vegetables in human nutrition. I. Seibold, Ronald L.
QP144.V44C47 1994
613.2′6—dc20 93-48257
CIP

Printed in the United States of America

Published by Keats Publishing, Inc.
27 Pine Street (Box 876)
New Canaan, Connecticut 06840-0876

Dedicated to Charles F. Schnabel, Sr. and George O. Kohler, pioneers of the modern use of cereal grass.

Contents

PREFACE

The Wilderness Community Education Foundation (WCEF) was established to support the development of sustainable agriculture and communities. WCEF is a part of a family of such organizations, companies and individuals located near Lawrence, Kansas.

Lawrence lies in the heart of the Kansas River Valley. The modern use of wheat, barley, rye, and oat grasses as nutritional foods for humans began in this area over 50 years ago.

Here Charles Schnabel, George Kohler and other scientists generated an extensive body of research on cereal grasses and the nutrients they provide. The Kansas River Valley soils are still among the most fertile in the world, but the negative impact of misguided agricultural practices adopted over the past thirty-five years is increasingly apparent.

The WCEF family is in the process of making dramatic changes in the land use practices of the Kansas River Valley. People associated with WCEF-related organizations share a common vision for the future. This vision is becoming a reality for those companies and individuals who use no herbicides or pesticides in growing food crops. Land is being weaned away from chemical fertilizers, and instead is being enriched by time-proven crop rotations of red clover, alfalfa and other legumes. Grasslands on bluffs, pasture lands and greenbelts are beginning to be returned to the native plants of the Kansas prairie. Communities are being planned around commonly-owned green spaces, facilities and enterprises.

The New Green Revolution happening in the Kansas River Valley is part of a planetary change in human activity and awareness. Its roots are in our collective subconscious mind. Each person who makes life choices toward this new vision of sustainable community life shares in our progress.

Like the New Green Revolution, this book is a group effort. It is a report on the research carried out by medical doctors and health scientists throughout the world. We would like to particularly acknowledge the contribution of Dr. George Kohler. His important research in the area of cereal grass and green food nutrition spans five decades. His suggestions were very helpful to us in compiling this information.

Writing the book was also a collective effort. The major credit for reviewing the literature, compiling the great volume of research material, and writing the early drafts goes to Lea Steele. She received editorial support from many others.

Author and wheat grass enthusiast, David Ding, of Petaling Jaya, Malyasia helped make the presentation easier to follow for Asians and will translate the book into Chinese.

Medical anthropologist and author John Heinerman reviewed the manuscript, checking for consistency and adherence to scientific fact and conclusion. Colette Roth provided many of the charts and graphs and coordinated the publishing process. Steve Malone and Bob Hoffman reviewed the text and provided many helpful suggestions.

Jerry Thomas edited the final draft for continuity and readability, making the information more understandable. Finally, my own name appears on the cover as coordinator of this project.

Everyone involved now has a renewed understanding of the critical importance of "eating more green." We hope that those who read the information in this book will find it helpful in improving their own health and that of their loved ones.

Ron Seibold
Lawrence, Kansas
November 1, 1990

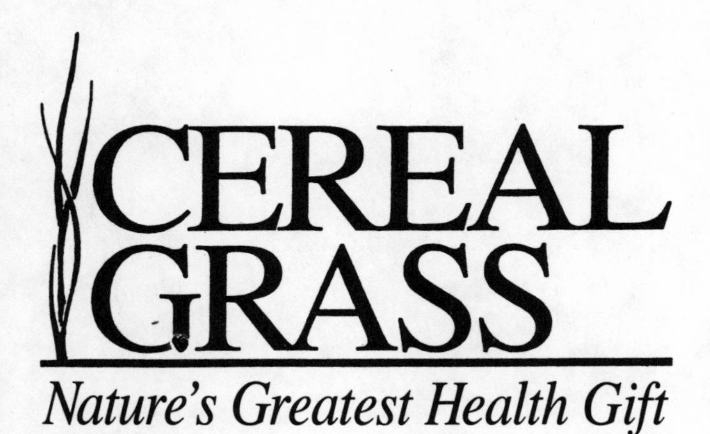
CEREAL
GRASS
Nature's Greatest Health Gift

Introduction

Cereal Grass has been around for a long time—thousands of years. Human consumption of wheat grass and other cereal grasses has increased dramatically in the last ten years, but most people have no idea of what cereal grass really is. Many of those who **have** heard of wheat grass or barley grass are puzzled about their purpose in the diet. Nowadays many people view with suspicion anything labelled with the word **grass** as a commodity for human consumption.

We see a need for a complete source of information on this food. And so, on one level, this book attempts to provide all of the information currently available about cereal grasses.

Wheat grass is, as the name suggests, the young grass stage of the wheat plant. Given soil, air, sunshine, and water, and left to its own devices, wheat grass grows into **wheat**, the familiar amber waves of grain. In its youth, wheat is a very dark green, leafy plant. Barley grass is the young grass stage of the barley plant. Other cereal grasses include rye grass and oat grass. All look, smell, feel, taste, and, most importantly, have the nutrient and chemical makeup of green leafy vegetables rather than of cereal grains.

Young cereal plants were valued in ancient times. It has been said that people in the ancient Middle East ate the green leaf tips of the wheat plant as a delicacy. Bottled, dehydrated cereal grass has been a popular food supplement for people in the United States since the early 1930s.

Nutritionally, cereal grass is similar to a number of other dark green vegetables. So in a larger sense, this is a book about all dark green vegetables—**why** they are good for us, **which** specific nutrients they provide to us, and **what** human health and disease conditions they might affect.

Most of us go way back with green vegetables, for better or for worse. Although some of us do "love those greens", we have to admit that many people consider cereal grass to be the perfect green vegetable because it is the most painless.

Everyone from our mothers to the Surgeon General has told us to eat dark green vegetables every day. But most of us don't do it. Salads made primarily from head lettuce don't really count as dark green vegetables, so we generally go without. Either we don't like them or just don't go to the trouble to prepare them.

Predicting or measuring the long range impact of a diet low in green vegetables is difficult. But evidence from population studies suggests that the typical modern diet may be associated with many of the "degenerative diseases" which are the leading causes of long term illness and death in the industrialized world.

So in the broadest sense this is a book about health, disease, and the modern diet. We provide basic, balanced information about nutrition and how it may affect our long term health. Contrary to the old saying, what you don't know **can** hurt you.

Nutrition is really a very complex subject. A vast amount of money is spent each year to investigate hypotheses concerning the effect of diet on how we feel and function. There are plenty of disagreements among people who are considered nutrition experts. Add to this the countless "facts" and claims made by those less concerned with validating their assertions, and the picture can easily move from complex to overwhelming.

Most of the information contained in this book is supported by research conducted and verified over the last sixty years in the United States, and more recently in Europe and Japan.

We have also included material which is based on our own experiences with the cereal grasses. To minimize any ambiguity, we have clearly distinguished research information from anecdotal information as it is presented.

We have attempted to provide a review of the scientific literature on cereal grass and other green foods, and to present this information in a manner which is understandable to non-scientists. We have also tried to avoid patronizing our readers with the pseudo-informational, panacea-type style sometimes found in literature about natural foods and supplements.

PART ONE

AN INTRODUCTION TO CEREAL GRASS

"I submit that scientists have not yet explored the hidden possibilities of the innumerable seeds, leaves and fruits for giving the fullest possible nutrition to mankind."

Mahatma Gandhi

Chapter 1

What is Cereal Grass?

"There seems to be no reason why grasses, suitably prepared should not be consumed by man with great benefit from the standpoint of general health and especially the prevention of degenerative disease."

Charles Schnabel[123]

Grasses inhabit the Earth in greater abundance than any other land plants. A large number of grass species have adapted to a wide variety of climatic conditions and soil types. The native grasslands in the American West once totaled over 700 million acres.[45] For thousands of years these tall prairie grasses sustained the life of the bison, antelope and deer who roamed over them.

Jacob Bronowski, in The Ascent of Man,[13] describes the miraculous genetic accident that might have occurred about 8,000 B.C., producing the bread wheat plant. The cultivation of grasses and the harvest of their grains have sustained the human population for many centuries. Agriculture has made possible the development of many of the world's great civilizations.[118] Wheat was a staple food crop for Egyptians as early as 5000 B.C.[148] The goddess Isis is said to have brought wheat and barley grains to the people of Egypt from Lebanon.[61] Wild ancestors to modern wheat plants still grow along the Nile.

The principal cultivated grasses are the cereal grains—wheat, rice, corn, barley, oats, rye and millet. Wheat is planted on more acreage than any other crop. It is grown most effectively in "grassland" climates, which have the appropriate level of rainfall and include a cold season.[3]

When the cereal plant is young, it looks something like familiar lawn and field grasses. It is leafy and has a deep green color. For over fifty years, researchers have known that the cereal plant, at this young green stage, contains many times the level of vitamins, minerals and proteins found in the seed kernel, or grain product of the mature cereal plant.[122] Grains are appropriate staple foods for animals, however, because they are excellent sources of food energy (carbohydrates) and contain adequate levels of important nutrients.

Figure 1.1 Wheat Grass and 100% Whole Wheat Four

NUTRIENT COMPARISON (Per 100 Grams Dry Weight)

	Wheat Grass	Whole Wheat Flour
Protein (gm)	32	13
Total Dietary Fiber (gm)	37	10
Carobohydrates (gm)	37	71
Vitamin A (I.U.)	23,136	0
Chlorophyll (mg)	543	0
`Iron	34	4
Calcium (mg)	277	41
Vitamin C (mg)	51	0
Folic Acid (mcg)	100	38
Niacin (mg)	6.1	4.3
Riboflavin (mg)	2.03	.12

Sources: References 52 and 153.

All Cereal Grasses Are Nutritionally Identical

The taste of young cereal grass leaves varies slightly with the species of cereal plant, from quite sweet (rye grass) to slightly bitter (barley grass). But the **nutrient content** of these grasses varies with their stage of growth and growing conditions, rather than with the species of cereal grass.[61] Wheat grass and barley grass grown in the same field and harvested at the same growth stage are more similar nutritionally than two barley crops grown in different fields. This fact has been demonstrated in thousands of analyses run on all the cereal grasses.[47]

How Cereal Grass Grows: The Importance of Environment and Growth Stages

Cereal grasses, like all grasses and plants, pass through several stages as they grow to produce their seeds (the grain kernels). A specific sequence of growth events takes place as the cereal plant develops. Each stage is essential; the basis for each stage is the cell quality provided by the preceding stage.[118] Specific environmental conditions—temperature, nutrients, and moisture—are required at each stage.

Plant **growth** and plant **development** are not the same things. A growing plant does not necessarily indicate a properly developing plant, or a plant which will produce seeds. For example, wheat plants can grow rapidly at room temperature, but can not mature in the same way as wheat grown outdoors and exposed to appropriate seasonal temperature variations. The chemical and nutritional profiles of cereal grasses vary widely at different growth stages.

Figure 1.2 Diagram of Young Cereal Grass Plants

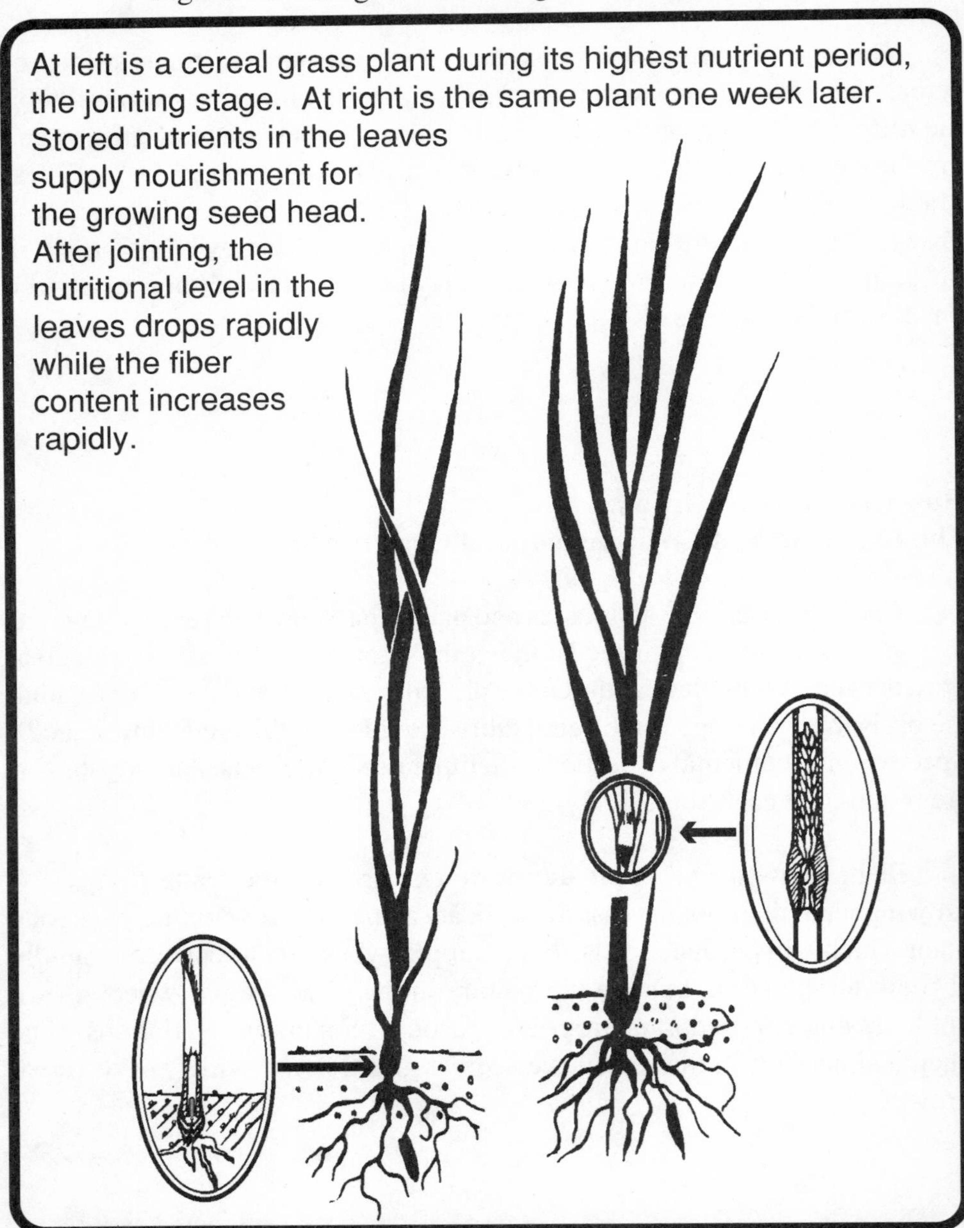

Cereal grass plants have a unique growth property. In the words of Dr. Charles Schnabel:[122]

> "In the battle for self preservation, grasses developed unusual resistance to grazing animals. Trees grew high out of reach, the cactus armed itself with spines, and grass plants evolved their unique property of jointing. In the early stages of growth they store large amounts of vitamins and proteins in the young blades. If these are bitten or pulled off, they grow again. Grass will give seeds to reproduce itself only if it is left alone at the final stage of growth."

Grasses have the amazing ability to provide food for animals, without diminishing their own ability to reproduce! In prehistoric times, this meant that a herd could graze on a grass range, then move on to another area. After the young blades had been eaten, the grass plant would recover fully and grow to bear its "fruit" or the grain seed, insuring the presence of the grasses the following year. In modern times, it means that when cereal grasses are cut before they reach the jointing stage, the plant can, with adequate rainfall, recover and continue growing to provide a grain crop!

The cereal grain kernel is not only the food from which we make our flours, meals, and other grain products, it is the seed which produces the cereal grass plant.

The climate and soil conditions in some areas of the American central plains are particularly well suited for the growth of winter wheat and barley. After fall planting and germination, the grain produces a shoot which appears above the soil in a few days. The roots experience active growth from October until the advent of freezing temperatures,[40] then grow very slowly through the cold of winter and early spring. The short blades of grass above the soil also grow in the fall, then become dormant through the coldest weeks of winter. The cereal plant's roots and leaves resume more active growth when temperatures rise in the spring.

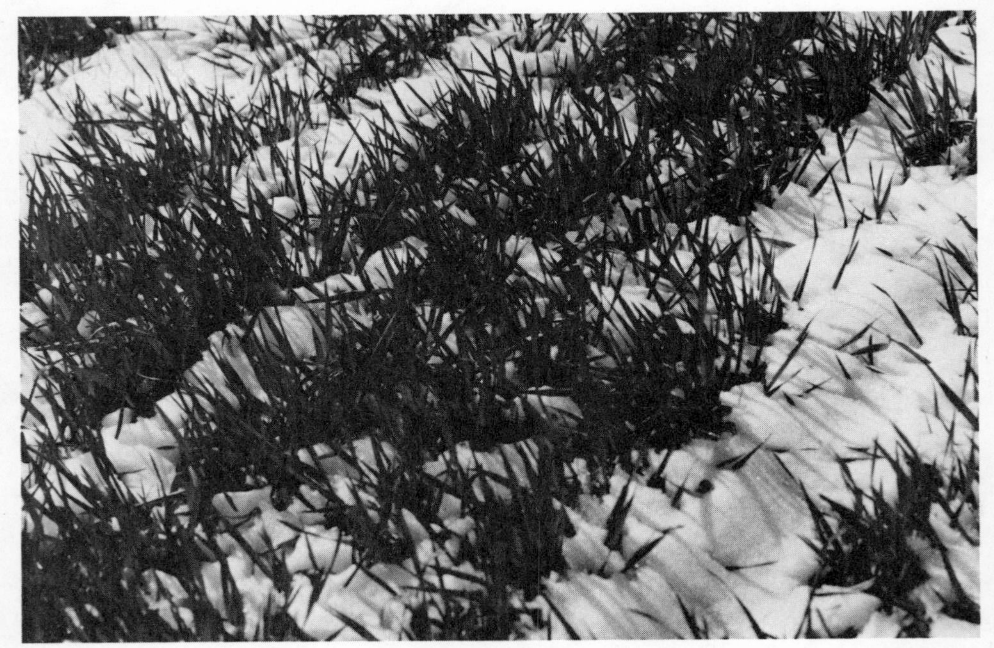

Most cereal grass is planted in the fall and is grown for about 200 days through the winter in the Great Plains of North America. It is harvested in the spring just prior to "jointing."

The young germinated plant is a factory of enzyme and growth activity. Photosynthesis in the young green leaves produces simple sugars which are transformed into proteins, carbohydrates and fats by the actions of numerous enzymes and substrates which were themselves produced from the plant sugars and minerals provided by the soil.[29]

Sucrose, the simple carbohydrate found in table sugar, is the primary molecule from which all organic (carbon containing) molecules are formed in the plant.[29] At the appropriate times and rates, sucrose is converted into amino acids (which make up all proteins), complex carbohydrates, lipids (fats), and nucleic acids (DNA and RNA). The degree of conversion of sugars to specific complex nutrients is dependent on the activity levels of specific enzymes in the plant. Enzyme activity levels are dependent on the plant's growth stage.

Winter wheat, for example, planted in a green house or in a warm climate, does not experience the environmental conditions necessary to produce normal root growth and leaf development.[40] Grasses grown in unsuitable environmental conditions may grow green leaves which are capable of producing simple sugars, but they lack enzyme systems which convert those sugars to the organic molecules necessary for the formation of a stem, stalk and grain seed.

The Jointing Stage: When Nutrients Reach Their Peak

Laboratory analyses clearly indicate that the nutrients found in young green cereal plants vary with the stage of growth, rather than with the age or height of the plant.[65] Chlorophyll, protein, and most of the vitamins found in cereal grasses reach their peak concentrations in the period just prior to the jointing stage of the green plant. Although this period lasts for only a few days, cereal grasses which are consumed as food supplements should be harvested precisely during this stage of the wheat or barley plant's development.

The jointing stage is that point at which the internodal tissue in the grass leaf begins to elongate, forming a stem. This stage represents the peak of the cereal plant's vegetative development;[65] factors involved in photosynthesis and plant metabolism would be expected to increase up to this stage.

After the jointing stage, the stem forms branches and continues to elongate. The chlorophyll, protein, and vitamin contents of the plant decline sharply as the level of cellulose increases. Cellulose, the indigestible plant fiber, provides structural stability for the growing stem.

Figure 1.3 Cereal Grass: Nutrient Content vs. Jointing Stage

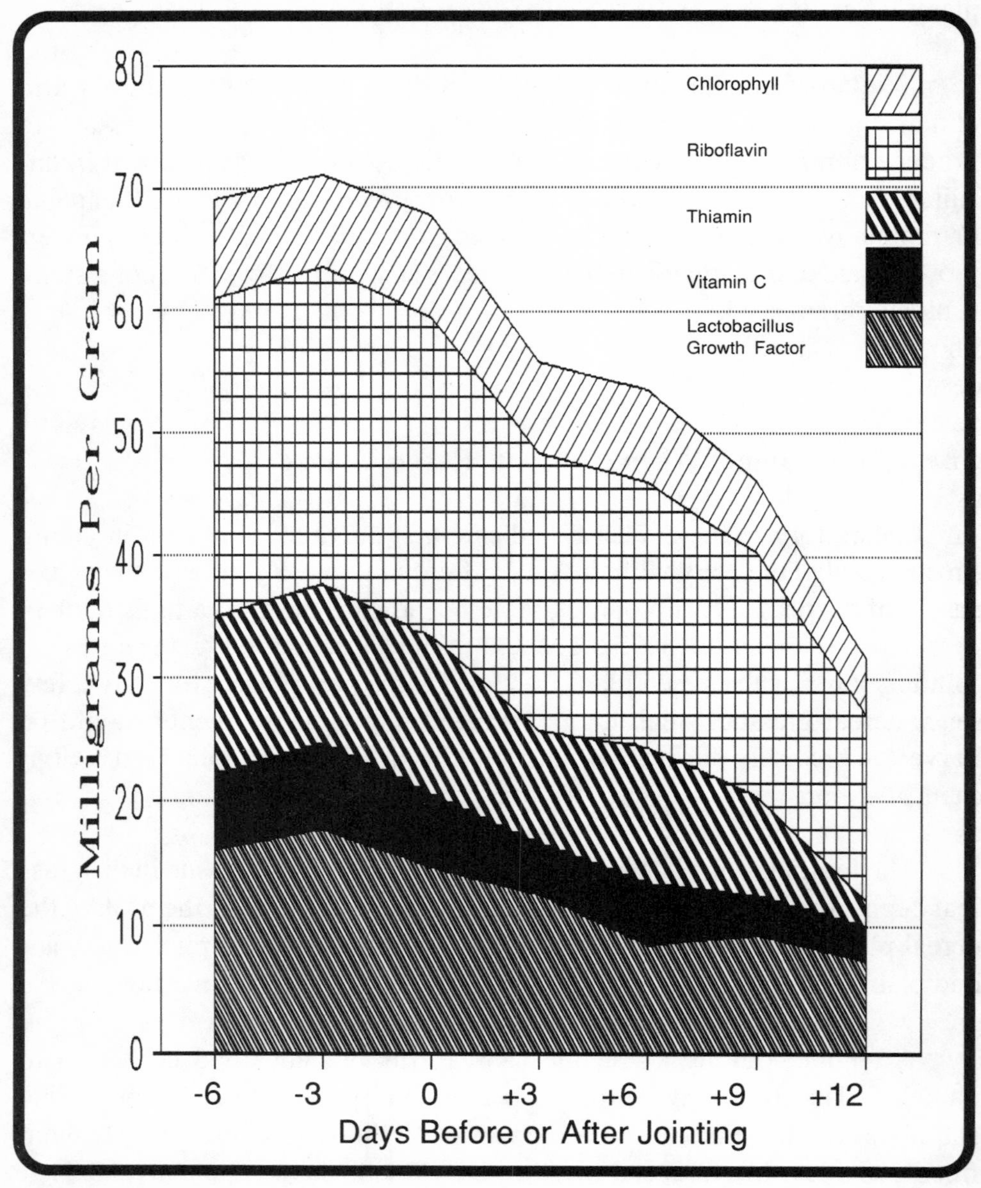

Source: Reference 65

Over a period of several months, the green leafy plants are transformed into golden stalks of grain. The mature cereal plant holds the seed grains which contain the nutrients necessary for germination and early growth of the young cereal plant. And so the seed-grass-grain cycle continues.

Home Grown Plants From Grain Seeds

It's easy to grow a grass-like plant from sprouted wheat grain at home. This plant is green and very sweet, but is quite different from the wheat grass described in this book. It is really more of a long sprout than a fully-developed grass. The plant is considered by many to be a good source of chlorophyll and an excellent detoxifying agent. This is the "wheatgrass" used by Dr. Ann Wigmore, Viktoras Kulvinskas, and many others in "alternative" health therapies for many chronic diseases. This plant has some similarities to the wheat grass plant which has been studied and used for the past fifty years. Both are green plants which grow from wheat seeds.

Indoor, tray-grown "wheatgrass" is usually ready for cutting in five to seven days. The sprouts shoot up quickly from the wheat seeds which have been germinated in water; no soil is required. The wheat seeds are placed close together and kept in the dark for several days. This is a standard method used for sprouting seeds.

This "wheatgrass" grows quite differently from the wheat grass planted in the ground to produce grain. Although it is a lovely and useful green plant, it does not develop deep roots, absorb soil nutrients, or pass through the growth stages necessary to produce the nutritionally potent wheat grass we are describing here.

The quickly grown indoor "wheatgrass" will never reach the jointing stage and will never produce a grain kernel. The simple sugars produced in the shoots by photosynthesis are never converted to the complex nutrients found in the leaves of the young wheat plant grown in the soil in cold weather. As a result, the tray grown "wheatgrass" has a strong sweet taste.

The indoor variety tastes so strong that drinking even small amounts (less than one ounce) often makes first time users nauseous. This sickening feeling is said to be due to the strong "cleansing" properties of the tray-grown "wheatgrass".

Certainly, there must be something in this plant which contributes to the remarkable recoveries reported by individuals who use the juice of this "wheatgrass" as therapy for chronic diseases. This plant and its juice is generally not consumed in large quantities, as is done with winter-grown wheat grass and its juice. Its value seems to be more that of a cleansing or medicinal agent than of a staple green vegetable food.

Why Eat Cereal Grass?

Dehydrated cereal grass is a **convenient whole food** which people eat as a green vegetable. There are many reasons why green foods are important, as will be seen in the following pages. We do **not** think that cereal grass should **replace** green foods in the diet. It is obvious that dehydrated cereal grass could never replace the flavor and satisfaction which spinach and broccoli lovers get from a big bowl of greens. But as green vegetables go, cereal grass is one of the most nutritious. And for those who have neither the time nor the will to eat more conventional green vegetables, a serving of high-quality cereal grass is extremely convenient. Winter-grown dehydrated cereal grass is "user-friendly".

Most of us grew up with our mothers telling us to eat our green vegetables. Today, many Americans do not like green vegetables and do not eat green vegetables, but feel they should. There is sort of a collective "green food guilt" which hangs over us. Even those who do like green vegetables sometimes think they cannot afford them or don't want to take the time to prepare them.

Figure 1.4 Nutrient Value of Cereal Grass and Other Green Vegetables

Vegetable	Serving Size	Protein (Grams)	Crude Fiber (Grams)	Carotene (IU of Vit A)	Iron (Mg.)	Calcium (Mg.)
Dehydrated Cereal Grass	(5 gr or .175 oz)	1.11	.82	1157	1.7	14
Spinach (raw, finely chopped)	1/2 cup	.9	.2	2230	0.9	26
Alfalfa Sprouts	1/2 cup	2.6	.85	-0-	0.7	14
Iceberg Lettuce (finely chopped)	1/2 cup	.35	.18	125	0.2	7.5
Green Beans	1/2 cup	1.1	.55	330	.45	31

Sources: References 98 and 153.

The preceding table shows the nutritional profiles of cereal grass and other commonly consumed green vegetables. The "green food" which ranks lowest nutritionally is head lettuce. Lettuce is tasty and crisp, but it is composed mostly of water! Those who think they get their quota of green foods from eating a lettuce-based salad are mistaken. Of the vegetables listed, the one closest to containing the nutrients found in cereal grass is spinach.

Perhaps one of the most important advantages of dehydrated cereal grass over some other green vegetables is the way most American cereal grass is grown. As discussed in Chapter 9, most of the produce we eat is grown using a wide variety of herbicides, insecticides, and fungicides which may contribute to our risk of cancer and other diseases. Cereal grasses can easily be grown without pesticides. The leading American supplier of cereal grasses produces them without chemical sprays. The consumer can read the cereal grass product label to determine the "wholesomeness" of the environment in which it was grown.

What Is Cereal Grass? A Summary:

Cereal grass is the young green plant which will grow to produce the cereal grain. All cereal grasses, including the green leaves of wheat, barley, rye and oats are nutritionally identical. These young **grasses** are, in their chemical and nutritional composition, very different from the mature seed **grains**.

Several growth stages are required for the development of nutritionally complete cereal grasses. Suitable soil, moisture, and temperature conditions are essential for the young wheat plant to pass through these developmental stages. The nutrients in the plant reach their peak values as they approach the brief, but critical, jointing stage.

The nutrient profile of cereal grass is similar to those of the most nutritious dark green leafy vegetables. The importance of green foods in the diet is now being validated scientifically. Because dehydrated cereal grass compares favorably with other greens with respect to both nutrients and cost, it is an excellent and convenient source of green food nutrients.

Chapter 2

Cereal Grass for People: Fifty Years of Research

"I have come to believe that the true medicine is young green barley and wheat leaves which are eaten by human beings as staple food. . . Such grasses as barley, wheat, rye, and rice too are as indispensable as the elements are."

—Y. Hagiwara[108]

Grass is the primary food for many species of animals. Some types of grasses make excellent foods for people as well. Ancient Oriental and Middle Eastern people are said to have eaten the young grass plants of wheat and barley. The Book of Daniel in The Old Testament says that King Nebuchad-nezzar (630-562 B.C.) ate only grasses for seven years. He claimed that his mental clarity, perhaps his sanity, was restored during this period, allowing him to again rule his kingdom.

The greatest ancient civilizations grew up in areas suitable for the production of cereal crops. In most parts of the world today, cereal grains such as rice, wheat and corn are the primary staple foods. Research on the use of the young green leaves of cereal plants has been carried out in the United States since the late 1920s. Dehydrated cereal grass became available as a human food supplement in the 1930s.

The Early Years: Animal Health Dramatically Improved With Cereal Grass Feed

In 1928, the concept of vitamins as essential nutrients was just gaining acceptance among health researchers. Vitamins A, C, E, and some of the B complex vitamins had been identified. Charles Schnabel, a Kansas City food chemist, was looking for a "blood-building material" which could be added to poultry feeds to enhance egg production and reduce chicken mortality. It was known at the time that chlorophyll, the green substance in plants, had some structural similarities to hemoglobin, the oxygen-carrying factor in animal blood. Reasoning that "green leaves should be the best source of blood,"[123] he began a search for blood-building factors in green leaves.

Dr. Schnabel first tried increasing the amount of alfalfa fed to chickens, but found that diets consisting of more than 10% alfalfa were harmful to hens. He then tried supplementing the chicken feed with various combinations of twenty vegetables, primarily green vegetables. All were "found wanting" and did not achieve the blood-building effects sought by Dr. Schnabel. In 1931, feeling frustrated and about to give up his search, he gave the experimental hens a "greens mixture," which "just happened to contain a large amount of immature wheat and oats." Chickens given a ration containing only 10% of this cereal grass responded dramatically. Winter egg production rose from the average 38% to an astonishing 94%! Not only were more eggs produced, but those eggs had stronger shells and were more likely to hatch healthy chicks. The chickens were free of the usual degenerative diseases associated with poultry production. Their combs were bright scarlet red, and their legs never lost their pigment. He reported that "even a child can see the bloom of health in the grass-fed hens, as compared to the alfalfa-fed hens, though science, as yet, cannot explain it".[123]

Dr. Schnabel studied many aspects of growth and nutrition associated with cereal grasses. He found that some soils were not suitable for providing high quality cereal grasses, and that the nutrients provided by these green plants varied with the stage of growth of the grasses. He gave the dehydrated grasses, an economical and practical food supplement, to his family of seven. As reported in the Buffalo Courier Express,[14] none of his children ever had a serious illness or a decayed tooth. He devised a plan to provide the hungry nations of the world with a high quality protein supplement derived from cereal grasses.

The "Grass Juice Factor"

In the mid 1930s, at the University of Wisconsin, Dr. George Kohler and his colleagues were studying the differences in the nutritional value of cow's milk produced at different seasons of the year. Although they thrived on summer milk, experimental rats and guinea pigs failed to grow and eventually became sick and died when fed winter milk. The higher nutritional value of the summer milk was found to be due to the grasses eaten by the cows in the spring and summer. Thus began research on the "**Grass Juice Factor**", a water soluble extract of grass juice which was responsible for this growth effect.[67]

Most of the individual vitamins were isolated and identified during the 1930s by scientists working to identify all the nutritional factors necessary for growth and reproduction in humans and domestic animals. Because the addition of green foods to the diets of test animals often produced dramatic growth and health effects, cereal grass and the Grass Juice Factor were intensely investigated. By the late 1930s, dehydrated cereal grasses were available in several forms for use as a human food supplement. They have remained on the market under a variety of trade names ever since.

At the University of California at Berkeley, Dr. Mott Cannon and his colleagues found that guinea pigs failed rapidly when fed a stock ration plus high levels of all the then-known nutrients.[18] When the researchers added standard food supplements such as liver extracts, wheat germ, and brewer's yeast to the animals' diets, the guinea pigs remained sick and often died. Addition of dehydrated grass or grass juice brought about dramatic recovery and restimulated growth in these animals.

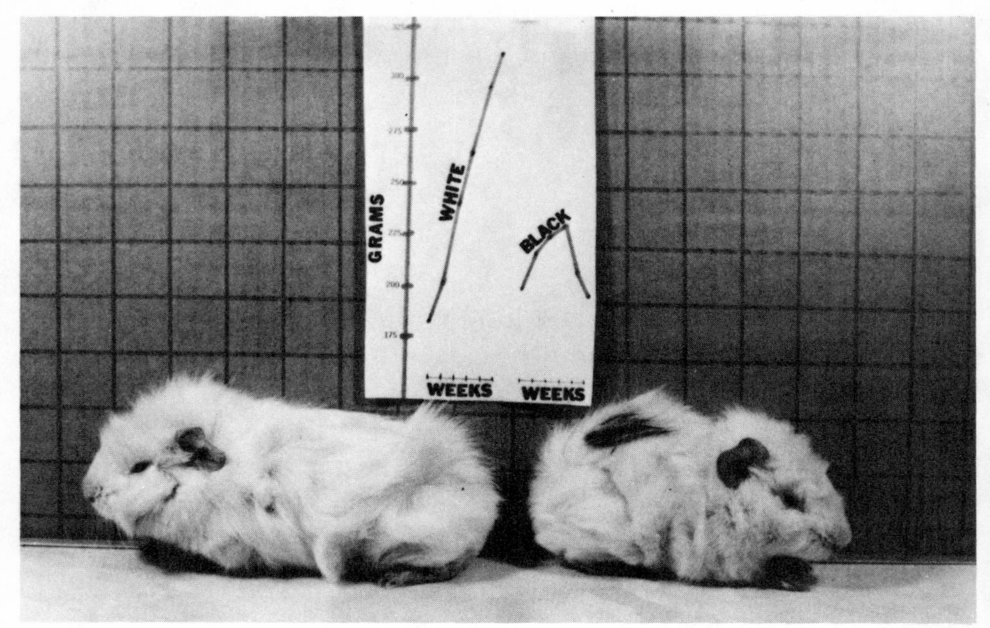

Typical of early studies, the guinea pig on the left was born smaller than his litter mate on the right. After five weeks with wheat grass added to its diet, the left animal shows rapid growth while the right animal (who ate only commercial guinea pig food) shows no net weight gain.

A large number of foods were tested at the University of Wisconsin to determine which of them contained the highest levels of the Grass Juice Factor.[113] The best sources were found to be dehydrated cereal grass, young white clover, peas, and cabbage.

In 1935, Danish researchers discovered vitamin K, the "koagulation vitamin". Because this nutrient was difficult to isolate in large quantities, cereal grasses were used in lieu of purified vitamin K—both for research and for medical therapy.[59] Folic acid was identified in 1938, and named for the green leaves, or foliage, which are its richest source. Food scientists were beginning to see that some of the health and growth benefits provided by the cereal grasses were due to essential vitamins and minerals which they contained. Other benefits, however, could not be attributed to known nutrients.

Cereal Grasses and Fertility

Research continued on previously unidentified factors contained in grasses. Earlier studies had indicated that cereal grasses enhanced the fertility of laying hens. In the 1940s, researchers in several laboratories discovered a substance in green plant foods which affected the fertility of several species of mammals. When injected into rabbits, this water-soluble factor actually induced ovulation! The factor was isolated from a number of sources, most notably frozen and powdered cereal grass juice.

The factor appeared to be most potent when supplied to animals in the spring and summer months.[11,39] It worked like a hormone by stimulating the pituitary gland to release another hormone which caused ovulation in rabbits, cats, and ferrets.[12] Spitzer and Phillips[134] then showed that a factor in green feed supplements improved reproductive ability and lactation when added to rat chow which contained all known required nutrients. When not given this green food factor, rats were less able to nurse their young, a characteristic passed to their daughters, even if the daughters had been fed the green food factor!

A significant number of reports show positive reproduction-related effects of feeding young grasses to mammals. Von Wendt[140] found that when human mothers drank the milk of grass-fed cows, their children developed more rapidly than children nursed by mothers who drank the milk of cows fed winter rations. This information supports Kohler's earlier work which showed that the Grass Juice Factor had a measurable impact on the nutritive value of cow's milk. And when fed to dairy cattle, young grasses produced noticeable increases in milk production.[11] A medical doctor in Kansas City[130] reported "gratifying results" using dehydrated cereal grass for pregnant patients who were at high risk for miscarriage.

Some of the fertility effects of cereal grasses may be attributed to their vitamin K content. However, the isolated factor used in the experiments mentioned above was taken from the water soluble portion of the grass extract, and so is clearly not associated with vitamin K, which is a fat-soluble vitamin.

Other Unidentified Health Factors in Cereal Grasses

Through the 1940s and 1950s, cereal grasses were found to contain a number of "factors" which had different health-related effects on animals. In addition to the growth and fertility factors, grass was shown to contain factors which support the growth of lactobacilli[25] and other beneficial intestinal bacteria.

Cereal grasses contain a factor which blocks the development of scurvy (vitamin C deficiency) which follows the feeding of glucoascorbic acid. This effect could not be duplicated by the feeding of vitamin C (ascorbic acid).[150] Other reports describe a cereal grass factor which blocks the formation of histamine-induced ulcers in guinea pigs.[64] Clinical studies conducted by Dr. Cheney at Stanford in 1950 demonstrated that green vegetables contain a factor which promotes the healing of peptic ulcers.[20]

By 1950, all the nutrients now considered essential to the human diet (with the exception of selenium) had been identified. But researchers continued to describe green food "factors" which could not be correlated with any known nutrient. In 1957, Ershoff again demonstrated the growth-stimulating effect of a green food factor for guinea pigs.[33] All cereal grasses produced similar results. Dehydration and pelleting of the green foods did not diminish the effects.

In 1960, the same laboratory described a water-soluble factor in alfalfa which improved utilization of vitamin A in rats.[34] This factor was shown to be distinct from known nutrients, including the carotenes. In 1966, Dr. George Briggs and others identified a "plant factor" in grasses, alfalfa and broccoli, which was isolated using the methods used earlier by Kohler.[82] This factor provided significant growth stimulation when fed to guinea pigs. Dr. Briggs' study is especially useful. It provides controls for nutrients (folic acid, vitamin B-12, zinc) which had not yet been identified when Dr. Kohler did his original work. To this day the "Grass Juice Factor" in young green plants, required for life and health in guinea pigs, has still not been identified as any of the known nutrients.

Cereal Grass as a Multi-Nutrient Supplement For Humans

Dehydrated cereal grass has been available as a food supplement for humans and animals since the 1930s. Before synthetic vitamin supplements were available, people took grass tablets to supplement diets which they considered to be inadequate. Doctors gave grass tablets to patients with nutrient deficiencies, or for specific health conditions.[22]

In 1940, Drs. Kohler, Schnabel, and Graham presented information about the nutritional properties of cereal grasses to the annual meeting of the American Chemical Society.[47] They reported that cereal grasses contain high levels of a variety of important nutrients—vitamins, minerals, and protein. These nutrients were found to be in highest concentrations just as the grasses approached the jointing stage of growth. In several thousand analyses of cereal grasses harvested at this stage, no consistent differences could be found between wheat, barley, rye and oat grasses. The Grass Juice Factor was said to be essential for the health of test animals given stock rations containing whole milk, iron, copper, manganese and vitamin C. Supplements of vitamins A, D, B1, B2, and B6 could not be substituted successfully for the Grass Juice Factor, nor could these supplements duplicate the growth effects provided by the factor.

The researchers went on to make certain observations which are still relevant today. They pointed out that about one third of the people in the United States at that time (1940) were unable to buy nutritionally adequate foods because of the high cost of foods such as milk and vegetables. Even those who could afford to buy adequate foods frequently did not choose foods which provided adequate nutrients. As a result, the researchers felt that a high proportion of the population was in a state of vitamin deficiency. Because the vitamin content of cereal grass was so much higher than that of vegetables commonly consumed, they suggested that the use of cereal grass as a human food supplement would be an economical way to provide those nutrients which were commonly lacking in the American diet.[47]

The dehydrated cereal grass food most commonly used was called Cerophyl (from the Latin **cerealis**, "of grain" and the Greek **phyllon**, "leaf"). Cerophyl was, in fact, approved as an "accepted food" by the Council on Foods of the American Medical Association in 1939.[10] The acceptance notice recognizes the value of cereal grass not only as a rich source of carotene, vitamin K and the grass juice factor, but also as a good source of vitamin C and the B vitamins.

During the 1950s, chemical and pharmaceutical industries began to play a bigger role in the production and delivery of American foods. It was the beginning of the promotional idea of "better living through chemistry" with a fertilized, crop-sprayed "green revolution". Agrochemicals began accumulating in our soils and on our food crops. Synthetic nutrients were added to foods and pressed into vitamin pills. As multi-vitamin pills became more commonplace, food-based nutrient supplements such as Cerophyl became less popular.

Contemporary Approaches to Cereal Grass Research and Consumption

The 1960s and 70s were times of social change and increased environmental awareness around the world. Growing understanding of our place in our environment and of our responsibility for the health of the planet, as well as our own bodies, spawned a revived interest in "natural" foods and therapies. In Boston, Dr. Ann Wigmore researched and rediscovered the value of cereal grass as a human food and therapeutic agent.

Dr. Wigmore, now over eighty, is an energetic and engaging woman whose vitality is in sharp contrast to her state of health forty years ago. As a child, she had seen her grandmother use grasses to heal wounded soldiers during the First World War. Thirty-five years later, when her own health began to deteriorate, she remembered her grandmother's remedies, and experimented with various grasses to improve her own health.

She began growing and chewing young blades of "wheatgrass" which she grew in her home. She soon recovered from a longstanding problem with colitis, which had been medically untreatable. She also fed the green plants to her pets, and wrote that "it worked miracles for their well-being". Her own energy level was vastly improved, and she began giving wheatgrass juice to her elderly and sick neighbors. "In a matter of weeks," she reports, "all of them were able to get out of bed, and they became more active than they had been in years."[145]

In 1968, Dr. Wigmore founded Hippocrates Health Institute, a treatment and educational center in Boston. To treat people with chronic degenerative diseases, she used wheatgrass and wheatgrass juice therapies, along with a diet emphasizing the use of green and raw foods. Many people who were "guests" at Hippocrates claim to have found, in the simple wheatgrass-centered therapy, cures for diseases considered by their physicians to be incurable. An account of one such cure is described by Eydie Mae Hunsberger in her book How I Conquered Cancer Naturally.

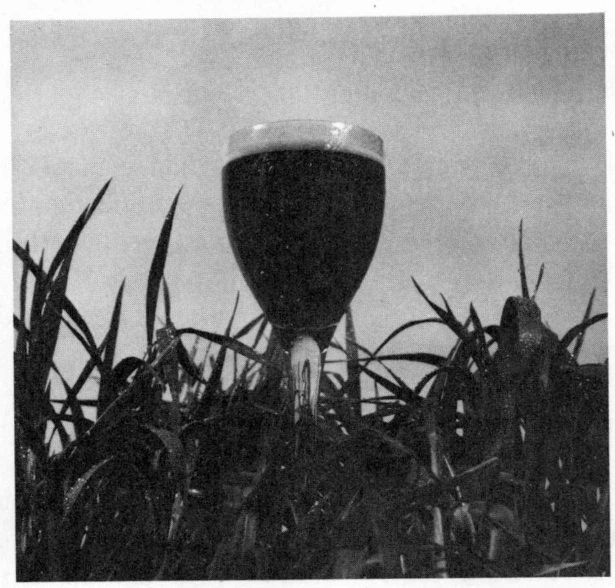

Shown above is wheat grass juice pressed from wheat grass harvested in the early spring after a winter of slow growth in cold temperatures.

Dr. Wigmore reports that the "wheatgrass" used in her program contains abscisic acid and laetrile, both of which may have anti-cancer activity. She feels that young grasses and other chlorophyll-rich plants are a safe and effective treatment for ailments such as high blood pressure, some cancers, obesity, diabetes, gastritis, ulcers, pancreas and liver problems, fatigue, anemia, asthma, eczema, hemorrhoids, skin problems, halitosis, body odor and constipation.[145] Dr. Wigmore's opinions are based on her experiences with her guests at Hippocrates. We have searched through the scientific and medical literature for information which might validate or repudiate her claims. Remarkably, a relatively large number of studies indicate that food factors and nutrients found in wheat grass may provide relief from many of the conditions she alludes to. No clinical studies have verified that such conditions can be cured by the use of wheat grass or "wheatgrass" alone.

Perhaps the most famous of Dr. Wigmore's "guests" is Viktoras Kulvinskas. He came to Hippocrates in 1969 at the age of 29, suffering from ulcers, arthritis, and migraine headaches.[117] Previously a computer scientist, Mr. Kulvinskas became co-director of the Institute after his own remarkable recovery. There he worked with the guests, and researched the health advantages of wheat grass and a raw foods diet. His book, Survival Into the 21st Century, has become a classic in the natural foods field.[75] He continues to work, write and speak out as an advocate of green foods and health awareness.

At about the same time that Dr. Wigmore began her work in Boston, a research pharmacist in Japan, Yoshihide Hagiwara, began to study the dietary benefits of cereal grasses. Like Dr. Wigmore, Hagiwara had developed a number of health problems over the years. After trying medicines and vitamins to no avail, he was able to improve his health with the help of Chinese herbs and a complete change of diet. Believing that his health problems were typical of many modern Japanese people, he began a search for the most health-promoting natural foods.[55]

Like Charles Schnabel fifty years earlier, Hagiwara found that "the leaves of the cereal grasses provide the nearest thing to the perfect food that this planet offers."[55] He also found, as had the American researchers in the 1930s, that the grasses of wheat, oats, rye and barley were extremely high in a wide variety of nutrients— much higher than the cereal grains produced by these plants. With colleagues in America and Japan, he carried out a number of animal and clinical experiments to determine the health benefits of cereal grass juices.

Although no nutrient differences have ever been found between the cereal grasses, the Japanese research has centered on barley grass leaves, which are readily available in Japanese barley fields. This research suggests a number of therapeutic uses for barley grass juice, including treatment for skin diseases[93] and ulcers, corroborating the research done decades earlier on the therapeutic value of chlorophyll and green vegetables. The Japanese research also demonstrated that mice, when fed juice extracts of barley grass, grew faster and had more energy than mice fed standard rations.[74] This research duplicates and corroborates a portion of the early work done by Dr. Kohler and others on the Grass Juice Factor.

Japanese research goes further to suggest additional, previously unstudied benefits of cereal grasses. Barley grass juice is said to lower serum cholesterol, perhaps by blocking intestinal absorption of cholesterol.[72] Two interesting proteins, P4-D1 and D1-G1, have been isolated from barley grass juice. These proteins may be connected to the previously unidentified factors in cereal grasses.

P4-D1 was shown to protect cells from ultraviolet radiation and a specific carcinogen. This was said to be a result of the stimulation of DNA repair by this protein. These results are preliminary, and have not yet been replicated. P4-D1 and D1-G1 have both been demonstrated to have antiinflammatory activity[73] when injected, but not when ingested. As with all cereal grass and chlorophyll therapies, these compounds are remarkably free from side effects.

Back in America, a limited amount of research has been reported concerning the potential anti-cancer effects of cereal grass. In a letter to Barron's Magazine, Dr. Arthur Robinson describes experiments carried out over a three-year period at the Pauling Institute. The effects of diet and vitamin C on skin cancer in mice were investigated. One diet, consisting solely of wheat grass, carrots, several fruits, and sunflower seeds, "caused a remarkable 35-fold **decrease** in cancer incidence"[116] when combined with high doses of vitamin C. Vitamin C, when given in high doses without the special diet, produced a five-fold decrease in skin cancer.

In 1979, Dr. Chiu Nan Lai, of the University of Texas Health Sciences Center in Houston, presented information at a meeting of the American Chemical Society[124] which suggested that wheat grass may have cancer-preventive properties. Using the standard Ames Test, she showed that an extract of wheat grass, when applied to known chemical mutagens (which cause cells to become cancerous), decreased their cancer-causing ability by up to 99 percent.[81] Later studies showed that several green vegetables provide anti-mutagenic protection from a number of cancer causing chemicals.[80] This activity was found to be proportional to the amount of chlorophyll in the vegetables.[79]

As we will see in Chapter 7, population studies indicate that the consumption of green vegetables may protect us from a number of diseases, including some types of cancer.

The idea of grasses as foods with specific health benefits is really nothing new. For generations, farmers have let their animals graze on the tender green cereal grass plants before those plants joint in the spring. We also see many of our pets eating only grass plants when they are sick.

Science is sometimes slow in catching up with conventional wisdom. Our mothers and grandmothers knew that to be healthy we needed to eat green vegetables. Their intuitive sense of the strength and health-giving properties of green foods has now been scientifically studied. A large body of scientific research now specifies **which** nutrients are abundant in green vegetable foods and **how** these nutrients can contribute to good health and disease prevention. Given the current status of our health, this information could not be more timely.

Cereal Grass For People: Fifty Years of Research: A Summary

The cereal grasses (wheat grass, barley grass, rye grass, oat grass) have been used as human food supplements since the 1930s. Scientists originally studied these plants as sources of blood-building factors. When, in 1931, it was observed that the nutritional level of milk fell when cows did **not** consume young green leaves, systematic research began on the health benefits of cereal grasses.

As essential nutrients were isolated and identified, the cereal grasses were found to be excellent sources of beta-carotene, vitamin K, folic acid, calcium, iron, protein and fiber, as well as good sources of vitamin C and many of the B vitamins. In addition, the cereal grasses were shown to contain unidentified factors which provide a variety of health, growth and fertility benefits to animals and to humans.

Laboratory research on the health benefits of cereal grasses increased over the past two decades in the United States and Japan. At the same time, the use of wheat grass as an "alternative" therapy for chronic diseases became popular. These two movements, together with the increased availability of suitably prepared American-grown cereal grass, have been responsible for a renaissance in the use of cereal grasses as human foods.

PART TWO

GREEN FOODS AND HEALTH

"Foods are the perfect preventive medicine agents. They provide a steady, but low-level amount of nontoxic therapeutic factors over a lifetime...varieties of factors that prevent many diseases simultaneously.

"As a disease preventive, a whole food is often better than individual compounds squeezed out of it. . . a food is a complex bundle of some ten thousand chemicals, breaking it down may simply dissipate its powers."

John Naisbitt[95]

Although all of us have long known that green foods are important to our health, most of us have not really known why. Green vegetables look good and taste good to some of us. We know they are low in calories. But mostly, we just know that they're **green**, and for some reason that seems to be good.

Before chemists isolated and identified specific nutrients, green foods were valued for their healing and "blood-building" qualities. Since the 1940s, a healthy diet has been defined as one which provides adequate amounts of all the known nutrients.

Dieticians and governmental agencies generally recommend that everyone eat at least four servings of fruits and/or vegetables daily. Of these, at least one should be a potent source of vitamin C. The other specific recommendation is that we eat at least one daily serving of a dark green or yellow vegetable. This recommendation is made primarily because dark green and yellow vegetables are rich in beta-carotene. Green vegetables, including the cereal grasses, are also considered excellent sources of iron, calcium, and folic acid. They are good sources of vitamin C and a wide variety of trace elements.

In this section we take a look at the specific nutrients found in the young green leaves of wheat and barley. We follow this with an overview of the relationship of these green food nutrients to diseases.

The first "nutrient" we look at is really not considered a nutrient at all by dieticians and doctors. Chlorophyll would be more appropriately labeled a "food factor", for it has never been shown by scientific research to be essential to the diet of any animal. But the value of chlorophyll as a therapeutic agent has been researched since the 1920s, and a substantial amount of evidence suggests that this green plant substance has many benefits for humans.

We then turn to an elaboration of the more conventional nutrients abundant in young green cereal grasses. These include vitamins and minerals, as well as extremely high quality vegetable proteins and fiber. This is followed by a brief look at the value of enzymes and raw foods in the diet.

Here again we emphasize that the story of wheat and barley grass nutrition is really the story of the essential nutritional value of all dark green vegetables. The importance of these foods in the diet cannot be overstated. The cereal grasses are concentrated green foods. It is important to include any of the dark green leafy vegetables in our daily diets.

Chapter 3

Chlorophyll and Blood Regeneration

Chlorophyll is the substance which makes green plants green. The chlorophyll molecule has the unique capacity to convert the energy of the sun into chemical energy (through photosynthesis), which the plant uses to make carbohydrates from carbon dioxide and water. Ultimately, all living things—plant and animal—derive their energy, and therefore their life, from solar energy through photosynthesis.

Yet, chlorophyll is not so unique in its chemical make-up. It is built around a structure known as a porphyrin ring, which occurs in a variety of natural organic molecules. The most interesting group of molecules which contain porphyrin rings are those involved in cellular respiration, or the transportation and consumption of oxygen. These include hemoglobin, myoglobin, and the cytochromes. Hemoglobin is, of course, the substance in human blood which carries oxygen from the lungs to the other tissues and cells of the body. The structures of chlorophyll and heme are shown on the next page.

Figure 3.1 Similarity of the Chemical Structures of Heme and Chlorophyll Molecules

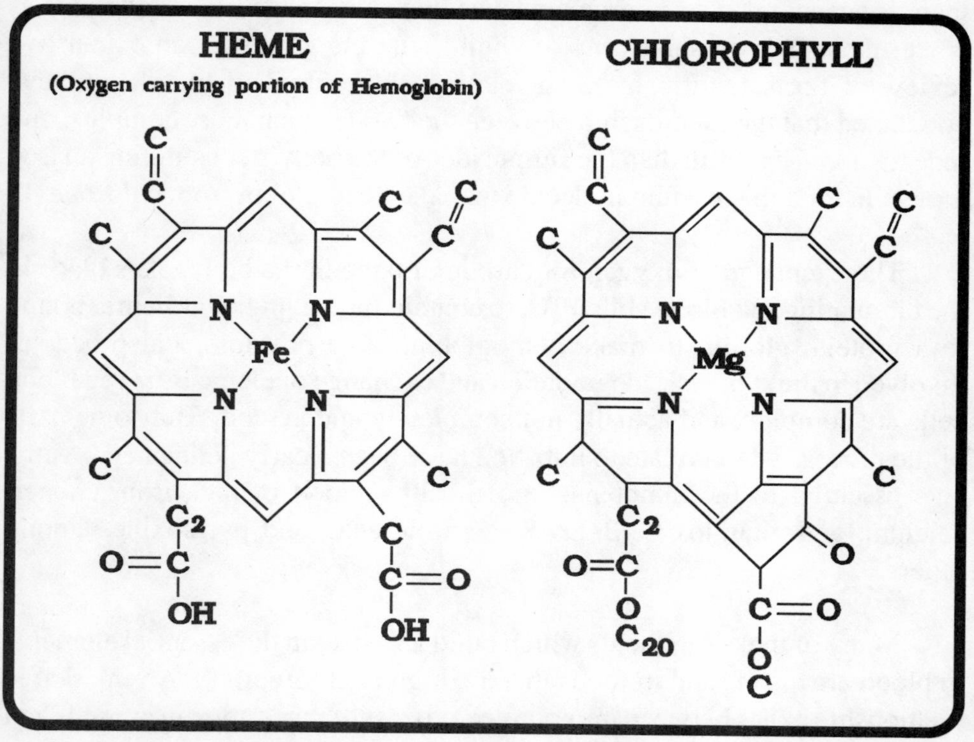

HEME

(Oxygen carrying portion of Hemoglobin)

CHLOROPHYLL

Obviously, the two structures are very similar. The most apparent difference between them is that the porphyrin ring of hemoglobin is built around iron (Fe), while the porphyrin ring of chlorophyll is built around magnesium (Mg). The chemical similarity between hemoglobin and chlorophyll was first suggested by Verdel in 1855,[19] and specifically demonstrated in the early 1920s. In the twenty years that followed, a considerable amount of research was done to see if the two substances were interconvertible in the body. We discuss this research in the following section. We would first like to point out, however, that the claim that chlorophyll and hemoglobin are directly interchangeable is oversimplifying the relationship between these two complex molecules.

Can chlorophyll, so abundant in the world around us, supply the body with hemoglobin, a vital blood component? It's an attractive idea. Certainly, there is anecdotal and research evidence that chlorophyll-rich foods such as wheat grass help in some way to "build" the blood. After an exhaustive review of the scientific research relating chlorophyll to blood, we have concluded that the relationship between the two is much more complex, and indeed more beautiful, than the simple idea of the body's substituting an iron molecule for a magnesium molecule to make hemoglobin from chlorophyll.

The exchange of oxygen for carbon dioxide in the body takes place in the circulating red blood cells. These contain the red pigment **heme**, bound to a protein, **globin**, to make hemoglobin. The physiological processes involved in the synthesis, degradation and exchange of elements in red blood cells are complex, and actually not completely understood. But some parts of the process which relate to nutrition have been clearly delineated. Nutrients essential to the maintenance of healthy blood include iron, copper, calcium, and vitamins C, B-12, K, A, folic acid, and pyridoxine, among others.

Many of the components which build and sustain the essential elements in blood are also found in foods that are high in chlorophyll. A remarkable relationship exists between the complex process of respiration in animals and the equally complex but very different process of photosynthesis in plants. In ecological terms, we know that the two processes are interdependent and are essential to the sustenance of all life on Earth. The inhalation of oxygen/expiration of carbon dioxide by animals complements the "inhalation" of carbon dioxide/expiration of oxygen by plants. The revelation that many of the elements of plant "blood" resemble and are in some cases identical to those of animal blood is not surprising in this context.

The young cereal plant, dependent on its own rich supply of chlorophyll for the work of growth and development, absorbs and synthesizes the nutrients it requires—vitamin K, vitamin C, folic acid, pyridoxine, iron, calcium and protein. These nutrients are also vital to the generation and utilization of hemoglobin, the energy courier of animal blood. The similarities between chlorophyll and heme are not limited to appearance and function. Chemists[89] report that the synthesis of heme by animals can occur in much the same way as the synthesis of chlorophyll in plants.[5]

For many years the general public and some health practitioners have considered green vegetables to have value as "blood builders". This opinion was reinforced by the observation that animals which ate only leafy green plants had ample amounts of hemoglobin in their red blood cells.[105] As described in Chapter 2, the similarity between hemoglobin and chlorophyll was the impetus for Charles Schnabel's groundbreaking research on the cereal grasses. As early as 1926, research suggested a possible relationship between the chlorophyll component pheophytin and hemoglobin generation.[121] Other studies indicated that feeding chlorophyll-rich foods to rats stimulated the regeneration of red blood cells.[125] Researchers were able to demonstrate that this effect was not due to the iron or copper in the green foods.

Early work done in several laboratories suggested that the relationship between hemoglobin and chlorophyll was not only chemical, but biological as well. In 1934, Dr. Rothemund and his colleagues reported that the porphyrins from chlorophyll could stimulate the synthesis of red blood cells in a variety of animals, but only when fed in small doses.[119] Drs. Hughes and Latner fed several doses and forms of chlorophyll to anemic rabbits in 1936. Extremely small doses of purified chlorophyll or large doses of "a crude chlorophyll extract" produced "a very favorable effect on hemoglobin regeneration". They suggested that "the chlorophyll is acting as a physiological stimulant of the bone marrow and is not really concerned with the actual chemistry of regeneration of the porphyrin".[58] This means that **components** of chlorophyll found in foods or when fed in very small purified amounts may stimulate the synthesis of red blood cells in the bone marrow.

In 1936, Dr. Arthur Patek reported the results of an interesting study. Fifteen patients with iron-deficiency anemia were fed different amounts of chlorophyll along with iron. It was already known that iron alone cures this condition, but Patek found that when chlorophyll and iron were given together, the number of red blood cells and the level of blood hemoglobin increased faster than with iron alone. No such results for this type of anemia were obtained with chlorophyll alone. As stated by Dr. Patek:

> "This study may serve to encourage the use of a diet ample in greenstuffs and protein foods, for it must be that over a long space of time favorably nutritious elements are absorbed which aid the blood reserve and which furnish building stones for the heme pigments necessary to the formation of hemoglobin."[105]

Intact chlorophyll molecules are not well absorbed directly into the blood stream of most animals.[6,66] So the extremely small amounts of chlorophyll shown to stimulate hemoglobin generation are probably all that can be absorbed from green plants.

More recent research[54] indicates that some porphyrins (ringed structures in heme and chlorophyll) stimulate the synthesis of the **protein** portion of the hemoglobin molecule. Thus, portions of the chlorophyll molecule may enhance the body's production of globin. This may provide a partial explanation of the effect of chlorophyll on hemoglobin synthesis.

Chlorophyll and Blood Regeneration: A Summary

There are many reasons why cereal grass and other dark green plants can be considered "blood-building" foods. The vitamins and minerals in cereal grass are essential to the synthesis and function of the components of healthy blood. But perhaps the most interesting connection between green foods and blood is the similarity in the structures of the two colored pigments, heme and chlorophyll. The biological relationship between these two molecules, though studied for over 60 years, is still not completely clear. It does appear, however, that small amounts of the digestive products of chlorophyll may stimulate the synthesis of either heme or globin or both in animals and humans.

Chapter 4

Chlorophyll as Therapy

"Chlorophyll, the healer, is at once powerful and bland—devastating to germs, yet gentle to wounded body tissues. Exactly how it works is still Nature's secret; [but] to the layman, at least, the phenomenon seems like green magic."

H.E. Kirschner, M.D.[63]

Although green foods have long been considered useful for their "blood-building" qualities, the chlorophyll found in green foods is itself valued for many other therapeutic purposes.

The leaves and green parts of plants have been used for centuries to accelerate wound healing. Among the ancients, the greenest plants were chosen for health remedies.[132] In this century medical scientists have found chlorophyll to be effective in the general fields of detoxification, deodorization, and the healing of wounds.

The power of chlorophyll as an effective deodorizing agent was first scientifically demonstrated in the 1940s. In the decade that followed, toilet paper, diapers, chewing gum, bedsheets, toothpastes, shoe liners, and a number of other products containing various amounts of green coloring and crude chlorophyll extracts began appearing on store shelves. In the wake of this "chlorophyll hysteria", a number of researchers began serious investigation of the therapeutic uses of chlorophyll.[131]

Chlorophyll Against Cancer

There is scientific evidence that chlorophyll and the nutrients found in green foods offer protection against toxic chemicals and radiation. In 1980, Dr. Chiu Nan Lai at the University of Texas Medical Center, reported that extracts of wheat grass and other green vegetables inhibit the cancer-causing effects of two mutagens (benzopyrene and methylcholanthrene).[80] The more chlorophyll in the vegetable, the greater the protection from the carcinogen.

That chlorophyll can reduce the ability of carcinogens to cause gene mutations has been verified by several laboratories in the last decade. Chlorophyll-rich plant extracts, as well as water solutions of a chlorophyll derivative (chlorophyllin), dramatically inhibit the carcinogenic effects of common dietary and environmental chemicals.[62,104] Ames testing shows that chlorophyllin neutralizes the cancer-causing action of mixtures of coal dust, tobacco, fried beef, red wine, and other compounds. In this capacity, chlorophyllin is more effective than vitamin A, vitamin C, or vitamin E against mutations induced by the same mixtures.[103,104]

Protection From Radiation

Green vegetables provide protection from radiation damage in test animals. This information has been reported in the scientific literature since the early 1950s. Early reports showed that certain vegetables significantly reduced mortality in rats exposed to lethal doses of X-rays.[133] Dark green broccoli offered more protection than the lighter green cabbage. In a later study, the same vegetables were shown to reduce the damage caused by radiation.[17] These protective effects were more pronounced when even darker green vegetables such as mustard greens and alfalfa leaves were used. When two or more of the green vegetables were fed together, the positive resistance to radiation was greatest.

Chlorophyll Against Germs

During the 1950s, many laboratories tested chlorophyll's power to kill germs. The consensus of these reports was that, for the most part, chlorophyll is bacteriostatic, and only slightly bacteriocidal. This means that chlorophyll limits the growth of many types of germs not by directly killing them, but by providing an environment which interferes with their growth. It is particularly effective against anaerobic bacteria, those which do not require oxygen.[131]

Dentists and physicians have successfully used chlorophyll to control mouth infections such as pyorrhea and Vincent's angina. Chlorophyll solutions provide significant relief of pain, reduction of inflammation, and the control of odor for patients with serious mouth diseases.[49]

There are several reported cases of the successful use of chlorophyll for bacterial endocarditis, an infection of the tissue surrounding the heart.[132] Chlorophyll has also been used successfully to treat chronic and acute sinusitis, vaginal infections, and chronic rectal lesions.[49]

Chlorophyll the Healer

Topical therapy refers to the use of a healing agent on the skin or other body surface. The number of surface conditions in which chlorophyll has been successfully used would be unbelievable were they not so well documented. And chlorophyll therapy provides an excellent bonus. In hundreds of experiments and trials on humans and test animals, chlorophyll therapy has always been shown to have **no toxic side effects**. Not just low toxicity, **NO toxicity**--whether ingested, injected or rubbed onto a surface.[132] This fact alone makes chlorophyll one of the most unique therapeutic substances known to medical science.

Chlorophyll heals wounds. The ideal wound treatment stimulates repair of damaged tissues and inhibits the growth of bacteria.[19] Chlorophyll does both! Even crude preparations of chlorophyll are effective in stimulating the growth of healthy granuloma tissue and fibroblasts—both on actual wounds and in laboratory cultures.[131]

In addition, the foul odors associated with surface wounds and ulcers rapidly disappear following chlorophyll application.[49] The medical literature is replete with reports demonstrating these effects. Surface wounds and sores due to surgery, compound fractures, osteomyelitis (bone inflammation), decubitus (bed sores), and routine cuts and scrapes all show fast and dramatic improvement with the topical use of chlorophyll. Chlorophyll therapy has saved limbs from amputation. Chlorophyll is also known to reduce the itching, pain and local irritation of surface wounds.[131]

Burns caused by heat, chemicals, and radiation also heal faster with chlorophyll therapy, whether or not they are infected. Chlorophyll was used to prolong the survival of skin grafts before the development of the immune-suppressing drugs which are now used.

The action of chlorophyll on wounds has a unique feature. Most medicines become less effective with repeated use. In contrast, an initial application of chlorophyll makes a wound more sensitive to its healing benefits with repeated use.[131]

Dr. G.H. Collings considered chlorophyll to "have the most constant and marked effect of all agents for stimulating cell proliferation and tissue repair".[131] Collings demonstrated that the healing time of wounds is shorter with chlorophyll therapy than with penicillin, vitamin D, sulfanilamide, or no treatment.[26]

Chlorophyll also accelerates wound healing by reducing hemagglutination and inflammation. When a tissue is injured, foreign substances in the blood generally cause blood cells to clump together. This limits the amount of nutrients available for repair of the injured tissue. When chlorophyll is administered to a wound, this clumping is reduced, so the lag time associated with tissue repair is shortened.[120] Chlorophyll decreases swelling by reducing the synthesis of fibrin (the protein associated with blood clot formation).[90,91] This gives chlorophyll a mild blood thinning, or heparin-like property, which can enhance the effectiveness of local immune defenses.

Chlorophyll has also been shown to be extremely effective in speeding the healing of peptic ulcers, wounds which develop internally in the gastro-intestinal tract. Several studies document the use of chlorophyll in the treatment of ulcers resistant to more conventional therapies. The results are quite impressive. In the Offenkrantz study, 20 of the 27 patients with chronic ulcers were relieved of pain and other symptoms in 24 to 72 hours.[99] Complete healing of the damaged tissues, as demonstrated by X-ray examination, occurred in 20 of 24 cases within two to seven weeks. These reports include case descriptions of dramatic recoveries from severe, long standing problems.

Other intestinal diseases have also been effectively treated with chlorophyll. Rafsky and Krieger[111] report positive results obtained with the use of rectal implants of chlorophyll solutions for the treatment of a variety of diseases of the colon including spastic colitis, sigmoiditis, and ulcerative colitis. The majority of the patients in the study showed definite improvement. Chlorophyll appears to alter the metabolism of colonic bacteria. Its use is associated with reduced formation of skatole, a substance formed by the bacterial breakdown of proteins.[131]

European investigators report preliminary favorable results in the use of chlorophyll in the treatment of pancreatitis. The chlorophyll is thought to influence several enzymatic reactions which complicate this disease.[21]

Chlorophyll and Intestinal Regularity

Researchers observed a side benefit when chlorophyll was used to treat peptic ulcers. Chlorophyll tended to "promote regularity" in the patients studied.[99] According to several investigators, chlorophyll did not act simply to stimulate bowel activity, as does a laxative. Rather, it promoted bowel **regularity**, stimulating bowel action only when that action was sluggish.

The same effect was noted in a 1980 study of the use of chlorophyllin (a water soluble chlorophyll derivative) to reduce body and fecal odors in a geriatric nursing care facility.[151] It was found that chlorophyll did reduce offensive odors, as anticipated, but also that it promoted regular bowel movements in these patients. Chlorophyll use also reduced the amount of intestinal gas experienced by the patients. And, as chlorophyll has no toxic side effects, the "gratifyingly good results" obtained made it preferable to the use of "drastic laxatives".

Green plants are still used as healing agents by traditional health practitioners throughout the world. But chlorophyll is used in a rather limited way in our modern medical system. The enthusiasm with which chlorophyll was once studied subsided with the development of antibiotics and steroid drugs. Dr. S. A. Chernomosky, in a 1988 review article in the New Jersey Medical Journal, states that the treatment of patients with slow-healing wounds is still problematic, and that the increased use of chlorophyll compounds may offer a useful alternative in this area.[21]

Today, chlorophyll tablets are routinely used by patients to deodorize the surfaces and contents of colostomies. Chlorophyll is also administered to incontinent patients to reduce odors in health care facilities.[151] Topical chlorophyll ointments and solutions for healing and deodorizing wounds are still available, as are chlorophyll-containing toothpastes and chewing gums.

The therapeutic qualities of this natural green pigment are still something of a well-kept secret in our modern society. Yet, many of us have an intuitive sense of the soothing feeling and healing effects associated with the color green. We feel it as we care for our house plants, walk on the grass in our parks, or see the new leaf buds sprouting from a tree branch in the spring.

Chlorophyll as Therapy: A Summary

Healing has been associated with the color green throughout history. Prior to the widespread use of antibiotic drugs, the green pigment chlorophyll was intensively investigated for its ability to heal and deodorize wounds of the skin and of internal body surfaces. The effectiveness of chlorophyll in wound healing is due to its ability to stimulate the growth of new cells while limiting the growth of bacteria. Chlorophyll therapy has no toxic side effects.

There is evidence which suggests that green foods may inhibit the damage caused to cells by X-radiation. Foods highest in chlorophyll provide the most protection.

Investigators in recent years have demonstrated that chlorophyll and its derivatives reverse the mutagenic capacity of some cancer-causing chemicals. Work in this area may provide future applications of a therapeutic role for chlorophyll.

Chapter 5

The Nutrients in Dehydrated Cereal Grass

> "It is one of those anomalies of nature and man that the countries with the highest rates of vitamin A deficient blindness are among the perennially greenest of the world, but the nutritious green leaves do not find their way into the mouth of the small child."
>
> Devadas[28]

Walk into any health food store or drug store and you might feel overwhelmed by the number of nutrient supplements displayed there. All of the vitamins, minerals, and amino acids are available individually and in creative combinations with other supplements. In those ubiquitous displays we can find combinations to build muscles, reduce stress, grow fuller hair and raise energy levels. The most popular supplements are the multiple vitamin/mineral combinations which supply at least the U.S. Recommended Daily Allowance (RDA) of all the known vitamins, plus a few of the minerals.

Surrounded by multitudes of "natural" supplements and remedies, it is easy to overlook the obvious. In nature, there is no such thing as 2000 mg. of calcium or vitamin C isolated into a single nugget. Furthermore, concentrated amounts of **all** of the identified nutrients are never found in individual foods.

Foods contain hundreds of compounds which interact with each other in the foods themselves and in our digestive tracts and bloodstreams. The combinations of nutrients and other factors found in foods bear little resemblance to those found in the supplement pills in the health food stores, and are many times more complex. Low-dose supplements may fill some nutrient gaps, and mega-dose supplements may have therapeutic value, but neither can come close to replacing our need for food nutrition.

The research described in Chapter 2 provides a good example. For over fifty years, the beneficial effects of adding cereal grasses to the rations of test animals could not be duplicated by adding any or all of the known isolated chemical components of those foods. The results of many studies which demonstrate the value of green vegetables in the prevention of human diseases cannot be explained in terms of the individual nutrients they are known to contain.

Why Wheat and Barley Grasses?

The cereal grass promotional literature of the 1950s claimed that cereal grasses contain every nutrient known to be required by humans except vitamin D, which is made in the skin. Contemporary laboratory analyses show that a wide variety of nutrients **are** contained in dehydrated cereal grasses. Some of these nutrients are quite concentrated, others are present only in small amounts. These nutrients are combined by nature to provide a uniquely potent food.

The following table summarizes the levels of known nutrients contained in the cereal grasses. The nutrient concentrations depend on the growing conditions and the growth stage at which the cereal grasses are harvested, rather than on the type (barley, rye, or wheat) of cereal grass analyzed.

Figure 5.1 Typical Analysis of Dehydrated Cereal Grass 3.5 Grams (7-500 mg. tablets or 1 tsp. powder)

VITAMINS:		PROTEIN	800 mg.
Vitamin A	1750 I/U	CRUDE FIBER	600 mg.
Vitamin K	280 mcg.	CALORIES	10
Vitamin C	11 mg.	CHLOROPHYLL	19 mg.
Vitamin E	1.1 mcg.	CARBOHYDRATES	1.3 gm.
Thiamin	10 mcg.		
Choline	1 mg.	AMINO ACIDS:	
Riboflavin	71 mcg.	Lysine	29 mg.
Pyridoxine	45 mcg.	Histidine	16 mg.
Vitamin B-12	1 mcg.	Arginine	39 mg.
Niacin	263 mcg.	Asparatic Acid	78 mg.
Pantothenic	84 mcg.	Threonine	37 mg.
Biotin	4 mcg.	Glutamic Acid	85 mg.
Folic Acid	38 mcg.	Proline	33 mg.
		Glycine	41 mg.
MINERALS:		Alanine	48 mg.
Calcium	18 mg.	Valine	44 mg.
Phosphorus	18 mg.	Isoleucine	31 mg.
Potassium	112 mg.	Leucine	57 mg.
Magnesium	3.6 mg.	Tyrosine	18 mg.
Iron	2 mg.	Phenylanlanine	38 mg.
Manganese	. 35 mg.	Methionine	15 mg.
Selenium	3.5 mcg.	Cystine	8 mg.
Sodium	1 mg.	Trytophan	4 mg.
Zinc	17.5 mcg.	Amide	10 mg.
Iodine	7 mcg.	Purines	2 mg.
Copper	.02 mg	Serine	85 mg.
Cobalt	1.75 mcg.		

Sources: References 64 and 153.

Many individuals have enjoyed the benefits of cereal grass for years. Research reports and consumer comments indicate that cereal grass is generally used for the following nutritionally related reasons:

1) As a convenient and economical way to enjoy high quality, non-toxic green vegetables.

2) As a concentrated food source of beta-carotene, calcium, chlorophyll, fiber, iron, and vitamin K.

3) As a good food source of the following nutrients: Protein, Vitamin C, Vitamin B-12, Folic Acid, Vitamin B-6 (Pyridoxine), and Other trace minerals

In addition, cereal grasses are used in laboratories around the world as a medium to support the growth of lactobacilli, the "healthy flora" bacteria which grow naturally in the human digestive tract.

Dehydrated cereal grasses have been used for over fifty years as a vitamin/mineral supplement. We won't attempt to provide a detailed account of everything these nutrients do in the body. There are many books which provide that information. Here, however, are the highlights of what is known about the nutrients which are found in abundance in the green leaves of wheat and barley.

Dietary Fiber

Many people who eat dehydrated cereal grass daily know only one thing about it—that cereal grass is one of the best available sources of fiber. It is one of the few fiber-rich food supplements which also provides an array of vitamins, minerals, and protein. The table below compares the fiber content of several well known fiber foods.

Figure 5.2 Total Dietary Fiber Content of High Fiber Foods

Fiber Food	(serving size)	TOTAL DIETARY FIBER Grams per serving	TOTAL DIETARY FIBER Grams per 100 grams
Dehydrated Cereal Grass	5 grams (.175 oz.)	1.9	37.5
Wheat Bran	5 grams	2.2	44.4
Oat Bran	5 grams	0.9	17.9
Whole Wheat Cereal (cooked)	1/3 cup	1.0	2.0
Prunes	1/2 cup	2.5	2.9

Sources: References 52 and 153.

Fiber is the general term used for the structural parts of plants which are not readily broken down by our digestive systems. It includes quite a large number of substances, some of which **can** be digested by the organisms which reside in a healthy colon. Digested fiber can be a significant source of food energy.[86,96]

The various terms used to describe fiber can be confusing. Many health claims made for "fiber" do not specify the type of fiber involved. But these distinctions are important. Different types of fiber have different effects in the body.

Crude Fiber includes the coarse fibers which are identified using older methods of chemical extraction. Those methods underestimate the total fiber content of a plant. Crude fiber consists primarily of cellulose and lignin, the least digestible fibers.

Total Dietary Fiber is the newer, more acceptable term. It includes all of the fibers contained in plants—hemicellulose, pectins, gums, pentosans, and the indigestible fibers cellulose and lignin. Total dietary fiber includes two **types** of fiber:

> **Soluble Fibers** are those which dissolve in water. They are found in foods such as oat bran, apple pectin, beans, and psyllium seeds. These fibers are currently receiving attention for their potential role in lowering serum cholesterol.
>
> **Insoluble Fibers** include hemicellulose, cellulose and lignin, and are found in whole grains and vegetables. Dehydrated cereal grasses are a very rich source of insoluble fibers. These fibers are best known for their ability to restore and maintain bowel regularity.

Dietary fiber has been extensively studied for the effects it may have on the serious chronic diseases that are called the "diseases of civilization". Because low-fiber diets are almost invariably high in fat and animal protein, it is difficult to separate the negative effects of a low fiber diet from those associated with excessive consumption of animal foods and saturated fats.

Colon cancer is the third most common type of cancer in industrialized areas of the world, but is extremely rare in developing countries. Because people in the developing world have diets higher in fiber than those in the more affluent nations, fiber has been studied for its relationship to the development of tumors in the colon.

Animal research indicates that **insoluble fibers**, such as those in the cereal grasses and whole grains, may reduce colon cancer.[30] The mechanism for this protection is the subject of much debate, but it is thought that the increased stool bulk and quicker colon emptying associated with the insoluble fibers may reduce the exposure of the bowel to carcinogens and other harmful substances.[86]

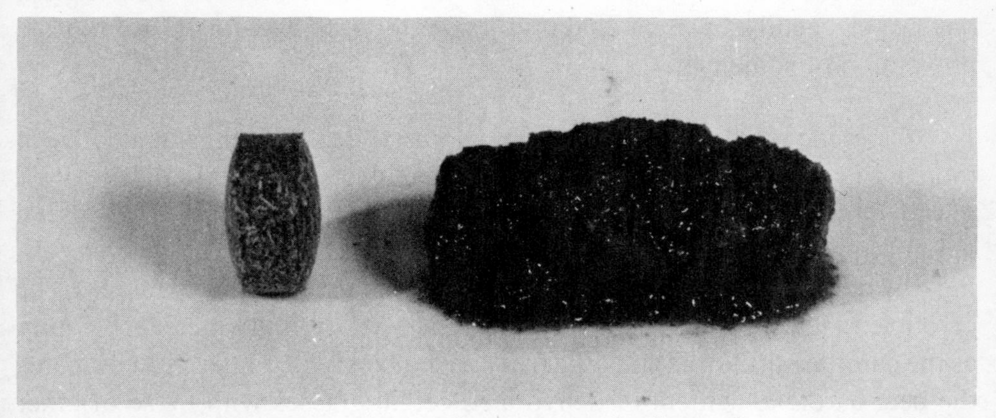

When placed in a teaspoon of water and allowed to sit for fifteen minutes, dehydrated cereal grass tablets expand dramatically, demonstrating why five to ten tablets are equivalent to a serving of other dark green leafy vegetables.

Dietary fiber has been shown to reduce blood glucose concentrations and the need for insulin by diabetics.[1] High fiber diets have also been studied and used for reducing blood pressure[2] and for weight loss. Insoluble fiber is often used to alleviate constipation, and is thought by some to be linked to the lower incidence of many gastrointestinal diseases (hemmorhoids, irritable colon, etc.) in developing countries.

The Food and Nutrition Board of the National Academy of Sciences, the National Cancer Institute, the American Cancer Society, and the U.S. Department of Health and Human Services recommend the generous intake of fiber for all Americans.[1]

Beta-Carotene

Beta-Carotene is one of the most popular nutrients being discussed these days. It is one of those rare substances which has received abundant attention from both the medical profession and the alternative health community. Beta-carotene has always been valued as a non-toxic source of vitamin A. It has more recently been studied and generally accepted for its role in the prevention of some cancers.

Carotene is a deep yellow-orange pigment. It is found in abundance in orange and yellow colored vegetables such as carrots and squash. Many **dark green foods are even richer sources of beta-carotene**, with the green chlorophyll pigments masking the orange carotene color. Generally speaking, the darker green the vegetable, the more beta-carotene it contains. The carotene in leafy greens is converted to vitamin A about twice as efficiently as the carotene in carrots and other root vegetables.[50,126] Figure 5.3 compares the beta-carotene content of dehydrated cereal grasses with those of other commonly consumed vegetables.

One of the primary reasons that physicians have traditionally warned against vitamin megadosing is that some people have overdosed themselves with vitamin A. The resulting disease is serious, and may even be life threatening. Preformed vitamin A is called **retinol**, and is found only in animal foods, where it is stored in the fatty tissues. Cod liver oil is loaded with it. It can be concentrated in our livers, too, and so is toxic in large amounts. The carotenes, especially beta-carotene, are converted by the body to vitamin A. But carotenes have never been known to be toxic in any amounts, although eating extremely large amounts can give an orange color to the skin.

Figure 5.3 Beta-Carotene Content of Selected Vegetables (in IU Vitamin A activity)

Vegetable	Serving Size	BETA CAROTENE CONTENT IU per Serving	IU per 100 grams
Dehydrated Cereal Grass	5 Grams (.175 oz)	1,156	23,136
Carrots (raw)	1/2 cup	6,050	11,000
Kale (raw, finely chopped)	1/2 cup	4,565	8,300
Spinach (raw, finely chopped)	1/2 cup	2,230	7,964
Summer Squash	1/2 cup	410	390
Broccoli (raw, finely chopped)	1/2 cup	680	877
Cabbage (raw, finely chopped)	1/2 cup	60	133

Sources: References 52 and 153.

The known functions of vitamin A are summarized below:

- Aids in the growth and maintenance of epithelial tissues and mucous membranes. This includes the skin and tissues which line our lungs, mouth and nose, digestive tract, and genital and urinary tracts.

- Essential for normal bone development.

- Required for normal function of four of our five senses (sight, smell, hearing, and taste).

- Required for the synthesis of DNA and RNA.[50]

- Supports normal fertility in both males and females.

- Involved in the synthesis of adrenal hormones.[126]

- Provides resistance to chemical carcinogens.[126]

Beta-carotene is an anti-oxidant.[16] Like vitamins E and C, it can bind and reduce free radicals, which are thought to cause cell aging and, in some cases, cancer.

Vitamin A and beta-carotene are required for several components of a healthy immune system. Epithelial tissues line all of the body surfaces which are exposed to outside elements. The mucous-producing cells on these surfaces provide resistance to infections and environmental toxins. They depend on vitamin A to remain healthy and functional. Vitamin A has also been shown to support the production of antibodies[42] and to enhance the immune response of polymorphonuclear leukocytes and other white blood cells.[8]

Moreover, both vitamin A and carotene have been demonstrated to reduce our risk of certain cancers, particularly those of epithelial tissues—skin cancer, lung cancer and cervical cancer.[70,78,100,112,139,152] The American Cancer Society strongly recommends a diet rich in foods containing beta-carotene.

Vitamin K

Vitamin K was discovered in 1935 by a Danish scientist who named it the "Koagulation" vitamin. It is one of the fat-soluble vitamins, one which we normally don't hear much about. This may be because vitamin K is synthesized by the healthy flora in the large intestine. Vitamin K deficiencies are rare in humans, except in connection with the use of some medications and certain disease conditions. **Dark green vegetables are the best dietary source of vitamin K,** which is usually found associated with chlorophyll in the chloroplasts of green plants.[50]

Vitamin K is best known for its role in blood clotting. Clotting is an essential function of the blood, and a rather complex process. The normal clotting of blood involves a combination of several chemical reactions, with each step dependent on the preceeding steps. Vitamin K is required for at least three of these reactions. The ability of blood to clot is crucial for the prevention of hemorrhage and excessive blood loss.

Vitamin K is also required for the synthesis of several important proteins which are not associated with blood clotting. Among these are osteocalcin, the sixth most common protein in the body, which is involved in bone metabolism.[50,126]

There was a time when patients undergoing liver or gallbladder surgery routinely suffered from excessive blood loss due to the clotting deficiency associated with a reduction in bile. That was before the discovery of vitamin K. In the 1930s and 1940s, before vitamin K could be easily synthesized, dehydrated cereal grass was given before liver or gallbladder surgery because it was the richest source of vitamin K available. Numerous medical studies reported excellent recoveries from this type of surgery when dehydrated cereal grass was administered.[115]

In addition, vitamin K has been successfully used for reducing excessive menstrual flow and cramps.[98] The vitamin is often given to newborn infants to prevent the hemorrhagic disease that is sometimes associated with the first weeks of life.[126]

Vitamin K deficiencies can result in spontaneous bleeding, failure to stop bleeding in response to slight injury, or excessive bruising. Deficiency of this nutrient can accompany liver diseases such as jaundice, as well as bile obstructions and pancreatic insufficiency. It can also accompany diseases which inhibit intestinal absorption such as prolonged diarrhea and cystic fibrosis.[126]

Medical therapies which can induce vitamin K deficiency include prolonged use of antibiotics, prolonged use of anticoagulants or aspirin,[50] and the internal use of mineral oil.

Normally, our need for vitamin K is met by the action of our intestinal bacteria, which synthesize it. However, any of the conditions mentioned above, as well as prolonged stress or the consumption of a diet very low in fat can increase our dietary needs for this vitamin. Research has linked excessive bruising and delayed clotting time, seen in over 50% of elderly people studied, to vitamin K deficiency.[50] Green vegetables, particularly the cereal grasses, are our best sources of vitamin K. Although synthetic forms of this vitamin have been shown to be toxic when taken in excessive amounts, natural vitamin K is completely nontoxic, even in extremely high doses.[126]

Vitamin C

Humans are one of the few species which cannot make adequate amounts of vitamin C internally, and so must obtain it from the diet. This vitamin is probably the most purchased and consumed isolated nutrient in the United States and Europe. It is said to prevent and reduce the severity of many viral infections, including the common cold. It has also been researched as a possible cancer cure or preventive agent when taken in large amounts.[116]

Scurvy, the disease which results from vitamin C deficiency, was once one of the most dreaded diseases in the world. Vitamin C is found almost exclusively in plant foods. The richest sources are the acerola cherry, citrus fruits and some green vegetables. Dehydrated wheat and barley grasses contain about the same amount of vitamin C as oranges on a per weight basis (about 60 mg. per 100 grams), and may certainly be considered a good source of vitamin C on a per serving basis.

Although vitamin C has been available and studied for many years, most of its biochemical roles have still not been identified. The major established function of vitamin C is in the formation of a protein called collagen. Collagen gives structural stability to connective tissues—those which surround and support our bones and ligaments, our skin and other epithelial tissues (see vitamin A). Vitamin C deficiency results in the inability to form collagen and the structural breakdown of tissues, including gums, bones, and blood cells.

Injured and infected tissues cannot repair themselves if the body is low in vitamin C, making this nutrient essential for resistance to disease (immunity), the healing of wounds, and the formation of scar tissue.[50]

Vitamin C is perhaps the best water-soluble antioxidant found in nature.[126] It acts with the other antioxidants, vitamin E, beta-carotene and selenium, to reduce free radicals, chemical substances which damage cells and cellular membranes. Free radicals are thought to contribute to carcinogenesis and the aging process.

Vitamin C can also act as a chelating agent, or a "grabber" of mineral ions. In this way it enhances absorption of iron and calcium. Inadequate vitamin C intake can result in iron deficiency anemia.

Several conditions have been shown to increase our need for vitamin C. It is stored in large amounts in the adrenal glands. Stress stimulates the release of adrenal hormones and neurotransmitters, and thus leads to the depletion of vitamin C.[126] For this reason, vitamin C (along with many of the B complex vitamins) is considered an "anti-stress" nutrient.

Higher than normal requirements for vitamin C have also been reported for smokers, elderly people, pregnant and nursing mothers, and for women taking birth control pills.

Folic Acid

One of the nutrients which is most often deficient in the American diet is folic acid or folacin.[50,135] Its name comes from the word **foliage** because one of the best sources of folic acid is dark green leafy vegetables.

Folic acid acts as an intermediary in all biochemical reactions in the body which involve the transfer of a single carbon atom between two substances.[50] It is particularly important in cells which are rapidly replaced, such as red blood cells and the cells involved in immune processes.

Several reactions involved in normal blood formation require folic acid. Deficiency of this nutrient is characterized by an anemia in which the red blood cells are abnormally large and improperly formed. Folic acid stimulates the regeneration of both hemoglobin and red blood cells.

Folic acid is involved directly in the synthesis of specific proteins such as hemoglobin and those containing the amino acid tyrosine. Folic acid coenzymes are also required for the synthesis of DNA and RNA, the "blueprints" of living tissues required for all protein synthesis. Vitamin B-12 is required for the activation of folic acid. Both nutrients may be stored in the liver.

Although many of us do not get enough folic acid in our diet, there are certain conditions in which even adequate levels of folic acid cannot be absorbed. Seventy-five percent of alcoholics have folic acid deficiencies.[50] Individuals who take birth control pills or anti-convulsive drugs may also be deficient in folic acid. Folic acid requirements are higher during pregnancy.

Although no toxic effects have been observed with high doses of folic acid, the U.S. Food and Drug Administration limits the amount that may be included in vitamin supplements because large doses of folic acid can mask a vitamin B-12 deficiency.[50]

Symptoms of folic acid deficiency include an anemia (megaloblastic) which cannot be treated with iron, disturbances in the gastro-intestinal tract, lesions in the corners of the mouth, and irritability.

Vitamin B-12

Vitamin B-12 is one of the more recently discovered nutrients; it was not isolated and identified until 1948, and was known for many years as the "anti-pernicious-anemia factor".

The primary source of Vitamin B-12 in nature is its synthesis by many types of bacteria. There is little evidence that Vitamin B-12 is made in the tissues of plants or animals. Healthy animals which are host to a large number of microbes are able to absorb and store this nutrient. Vitamin B-12 is contained, then, in a wide variety of foods of animal origin—meats and dairy foods. Plant foods are generally considered to be devoid of Vitamin B-12. For this reason, vegetarians who consume no animal products are often advised to take Vitamin B-12 supplements.

Surprisingly, laboratory analyses from the past forty years consistently show that **dehydrated cereal grass does contain appreciable amounts of vitamin B-12**. Laboratory tests show that a day's supply (ten grams) of dehydrated cereal grass contains between .24 and .44 micrograms of vitamin B-12,[64] or four to eight percent of the Recommended Daily Allowance for this nutrient. The B-12 found in wheat and barley grasses may be there in connection with microbes found in the soils in which the grasses are grown, or the positive flora (lactobacilli) which are known to thrive on cereal grasses.

Vitamin B-12 has many important functions, which are often related to the functions of other B-complex vitamins. It is required for the conversion of folic acid from the inactive form to the active form. It is essential for the proper formation and maturing of red blood cells and the synthesis of DNA and RNA. It is needed for normal growth and for the maintenance of healthy nerve tissues. It is also involved in fat and protein metabolism.[50]

The human liver can store up to a 6-year supply of vitamin B-12. Large doses of this vitamin are sometimes injected for a number of therapeutic reasons ranging from menopausal problems to a general lack of energy. The effectiveness of these uses of the vitamin has not been firmly established, nor have toxic effects been seen from high doses.

Absorption of vitamin B-12 requires the presence of a protein called intrinsic factor, which requires pyridoxine for its synthesis.

Pyridoxine

Pyridoxine is also known as vitamin B6. It is required for processes involved in the synthesis of a number of proteins. For example, pyridoxine is directly involved in the formation of the protein heme, which is the iron-containing portion of the hemoglobin molecule. It is necessary for the production of nucleic acids (DNA and RNA) as well as for RNA's use of amino acids to make proteins. Pyridoxine functions as a coenzyme, needed for the function of enzymes, in the body's use of carbohydrates and lipids.

Pyridoxine is essential for the formation of the neurotransmitters which send impulses through the brain and nervous system. It is also needed for the formation of antibodies—crucial elements in immune defenses against disease.[50]

Pyridoxine is water soluble, and cannot be stored in the body. The 1978 Food Consumption Survey showed that almost half of those people evaluated got less than 70% of the RDA of this nutrient in their normal diet.[50] Pregnant women and those who take oral contraceptives have a special need for this vitamin. Deficiency of pyridoxine is associated with a type of anemia in which the body has large amounts of iron. Insufficient levels of pyridoxine may also be associated with irritability, insomnia, and the formation of kidney stones.[50]

Cereal grasses are somewhat richer sources of pyridoxine than most green vegetables. Its presence in these green foods is important because it complements the presence of folic acid, vitamin B12, vitamin C and iron as a support nutrient for the maintenance of blood hemoglobin levels and a healthy immune system.

Iron

Most of the body's iron is contained in the hemoglobin molecule, the blood protein which carries oxygen to body tissues. But iron is also present throughout the body, and is known to be essential to a wide variety of enzymatic reactions. The major physiological uses for iron are these:[50]

- Central element in heme protein, essential for transport of oxygen and carbon dioxide throughout the body.

- Needed for the conversion of beta-carotene to the active form of vitamin A.

- Essential for antibody production.

- Required for the synthesis of DNA and RNA.

- Involved in the detoxification of drugs by the liver.

Our absorption of the **non**-heme iron in plant foods is facilitated by the presence of an acid such as vitamin C. Absorption of dietary iron is increased when hemoglobin levels are low, and reduced when our iron stores are adequate. Although iron deficiencies are rare in men, the majority of American women have been shown to have diets which provide less than 60% of the RDA for iron.[50]

Iron deficiency results in anemia, a condition characterized by a low concentration of hemoglobin in the blood and by paleness and abnormal fatigue. Insufficient iron is also associated with increased susceptibility to infections, inability to concentrate, apathy and irritability.[52]

Calcium

Calcium is the most abundant mineral in the body. The hard tissues—bones and teeth—contain ninety-nine percent of the body's calcium. The remaining one percent is distributed throughout the cells and fluids of the body. This relatively small amount of calcium is of huge importance in vital functions. Processes for which calcium is required by the body are summarized below:

- Combines with phosphorous to form the hard substance of bones and teeth.
- Essential for muscle contraction including the maintenance of heart contractions.
- Involved in the transmission of nerve impulses.
- Required at each step in the cascade of reactions necessary for blood clotting.
- Aids in the absorption of vitamin B-12.
- Needed for fat metabolism and the secretion of insulin.

In America and Western Europe, dairy foods are the primary dietary sources of calcium. In many areas of the developing world, however, only mother's milk is consumed. Studies in African populations show that the calcium supplied by a number of green leafy plants can be absorbed in quantities comparable to the calcium absorbed from dairy products.[36] Osteoporosis is uncommon in many areas of the world where dairy products are rarely consumed.[88]

Calcium absorption can be inhibited by natural plant substances such as oxalates and phytates. Oxalic acid is highly concentrated in rhubarb, cocoa and in some leafy greens such as spinach and Swiss chard. Dehydrated cereal grass contains only small amounts of oxalic acid.[10] Phytates are contained in the outer husk of whole grains. High protein diets are also thought to reduce calcium absorption.[50,88] Calcium absorption requires vitamin D and is enhanced by estrogen.

Osteoporosis ("porous bones") is a major problem for the elderly. It is thought to be a result of a prolonged imbalance between calcium absorption and calcium needs, resulting in brittle bones which are easily fractured. People of all ages, particularly middle-aged and elderly women, need to maintain an adequate level of calcium in their diets to avoid bone loss. Regular exercise can also help to minimize bone loss. Smoking and alcohol consumption contribute to the risk of osteoporosis.[52]

Protein

Protein is a part of every living cell. It accounts for over half of the dry weight of the human body. The protein contained in cereal grasses and other green leaves is a nutrition resource that has barely been tapped. Dehydrated cereal grass is twenty to twenty-five percent protein, making it higher than milk (3%), eggs (12%), and sirloin steak (16%)! Of course, as nutritionists know, all proteins are not created equal. But **the protein in cereal grass is superior to that of any other plant source**, and is even superior to that of some animal foods.[109]

Proteins are built from chemical building blocks called amino acids. There are 20 different amino acids which make up proteins. Healthy adult humans can make all but 9 of these in adequate quantities.[50,52] The remaining 9 amino acids must be obtained from the foods we eat, and are called **essential amino acids**.

In order for food proteins to be optimally used by the body, **all** of the essential amino acids must be present in suitable proportions. Proteins which meet this requirement are called **complete proteins**. Those which are deficient in one or more amino acids are called **incomplete proteins**.

Most animal-food proteins are considered complete proteins; plant proteins are usually considered incomplete. Vegetarians often combine protein foods to balance the different amino acids which are low in each. Grain foods tend to be low in the essential amino acid lysine, while beans often lack methionine. Eggs are believed to contain the most usable combination of amino acids.

Cereal grasses contain all of the essential amino acids in amounts which make the protein very usable. Unlike most plant proteins, these grasses contain high levels of **both** methionine and lysine.

Figure 5.4 Comparisons of Cereal Grass Protein to Ideal Proten

Profiles of Essential Amino Acids
"Ideal Protein*" and Cereal Grass**
Milligrams Amino Acid per Gram of Protein
Valine
Tryptophan
Threonine
Phenylalamine+
Methionine+
Lysine
Leucine
Isoleucine
Histidine
0 10 20 30 40 50 60 70 80 90
Ideal Protein
Dehydrated Cereal Grass
*Values established by Food and Agricultural Organization/Whold Health Organization

**Source: Reference 153.

The value of the protein found in green leafy plants is relatively consistent throughout nature.[109] Because the world has such an abundant supply of green plants—both cultivated and wild—scientists have investigated ways of using green plants as a source of protein in areas where diets lack adequate levels of protein.

The importance of adequate protein in the diet cannot be overemphasized. The amino acids in dietary proteins are used to build all of the proteins which our bodies need. Among the most crucial functions of proteins are:

- Formation of essential compounds including antibodies, hormones, neurotransmitters and enzymes.

- The growth of all tissues and the replacement of damaged tissues, including blood cells.

- An important source of food energy.

- Maintenance of electrolyte/water balance and acid/base balance.

The first item alone reminds us that it would be impossible to stay healthy or even to function without adequate protein. In many parts of the world there is an alarming rate of protein-energy malnutrition, especially among children.

In areas of the world where food availability is less of a problem, it is very difficult for anyone eating a reasonably balanced diet **not** to meet minimum protein needs, even when the diet contains little or no animal foods.[52] Some nutritionists now say that some people in the developed areas of the world eat **too much protein**. Dr. John McDougall, noted physician, author, and nutrition authority, warns that high protein diets may be the major cause of osteoporosis.[88] Excessive intake of **animal proteins** has been linked in several studies to an increased risk of colon cancer[76] and coronary heart disease.[53]

Nutrient Synergism in the Cereal Grasses

Dehydrated cereal grass tablets are **not** multi-vitamin pills. They are a concentrated combination of the nutrients found in all the higher quality dark green vegetables. As we have seen, the nutrients found in these foods work together to benefit the body as a whole. It may also have become apparent that the cereal grasses contain nutrients which support inter-related functions of our vital systems and physiological processes.

It is interesting, and rather amazing, to see how the variety of nutrients in the cereal grasses support the functions of other nutrients which are found there. A closer look at this phenomenon makes a good case for relying on foods rather than vitamin pills as sources of vitamins and minerals.

For example, vitamin C aids in the absorption of calcium and iron. Iron is required to convert beta-carotene to vitamin A. Calcium and pyridoxine help absorb vitamin B12, which is essential for the activation of folic acid. All of these nutrients are found together in the cereal grasses, along with others which support complimentary functions.

Healthy Blood and Circulation

Green food nutrients support healthy blood and circulation. Iron, folic acid, vitamin C, vitamin B12, pyridoxine, and protein are all vital for the formation and maintenance of adequate levels of hemoglobin and red blood cells. Chlorophyll may also be beneficial in these processes. In addition, chlorophyll, vitamin K, and calcium are all involved in blood clot formation and breakdown.

Detoxification

Dehydrated cereal grasses are perhaps most often consumed as fiber foods, and for their maintenance of bowel regularity. Their combination of insoluble fiber and chlorophyll make them excellent foods for this purpose. In addition, beta-carotene supports the growth and maintenance of the lining of the intestinal tract.

The mechanisms by which green foods provide protection from chemical carcinogens and radiation are not entirely clear. It has been shown that chlorophyll, beta-carotene, and vitamin C may contribute to this protection. The latter two nutrients are anti-oxidants, and chlorophyll may provide protection against DNA mutations in ways which are not yet known.

Immune System Support

Our bodies are constantly making and using immune cells. These cells are said, therefore, to have a high turnover rate. Cells and tissues with a high turnover rate are particularly sensitive to inadequate nutrition. The specific nutrients needed for the synthesis of immune cells and products include protein, vitamin A, vitamin C, iron, folic acid, and pyridoxine. Green vegetables are excellent sources of these nutrients. On a larger scale, it is thought that fiber foods provide some immune protection to the intestinal tract by reducing the amount of toxic material which contacts and penetrates the colon.

The Nutrients in Dehydrated Cereal Grass: A Summary

Wheat grass, barley grass, and all the dark green vegetables contain a wide variety of essential vitamins and minerals. These nutrients are combined by nature with high quality vegetable protein and fibers, to provide naturally potent foods. Green foods have been an essential part of the human diet for thousands, perhaps millions of years. Today, we are able to identify many of the specific nutrients found in green foods, and the reasons why we can't do without them. Even with all of this information, we may only be beginning to understand why green foods are so good for us.

Chapter 6

Enzymes and Live Foods

Among the health claims commonly made for natural foods and supplements, including the cereal grasses, is the promise of the benefits of **active enzymes**. Dehydrated wheat grass and barley grass do contain a wide variety of enzymes, but current evidence suggests that the health benefits provided by dietary enzymes is limited, at best. We believe it is important that some balanced information on this subject be provided.

Almost everyone has heard the word enzyme. People who are less familiar with the biological sciences tend to think of enzymes as sort of magical, living chemicals. In a sense, they are right.

All proteins associated with the human body, or with any living system, **do** something. Some of them form structures, like fingernails; others, like hormones, participate in chemical reactions. **Enzymes are proteins which stimulate chemical reactions between other proteins.** They are present in every living thing, and may continue to function long after the organism is no longer technically alive.

The reactions which enzymes stimulate are essential to the life process. It is estimated that a single human liver cell contains at least 1,000 different enzyme systems.[50] The total number of enzymes in our bodies can only be speculated on; the number of individual enzyme molecules is virtually inestimable. The same is true for any complex living system, such as a green plant.

Enzymes do their work by reducing the energy required for individual reactions to take place. In other words, enzymes make it easier for two proteins to react together. Enzymes themselves are not altered by the reactions they stimulate; they are not "used up" by performing their functions. They are catalysts. Figure 6.1 illustrates this principle.

Figure 6.1 Diagrammatic Representation of Enzyme Action

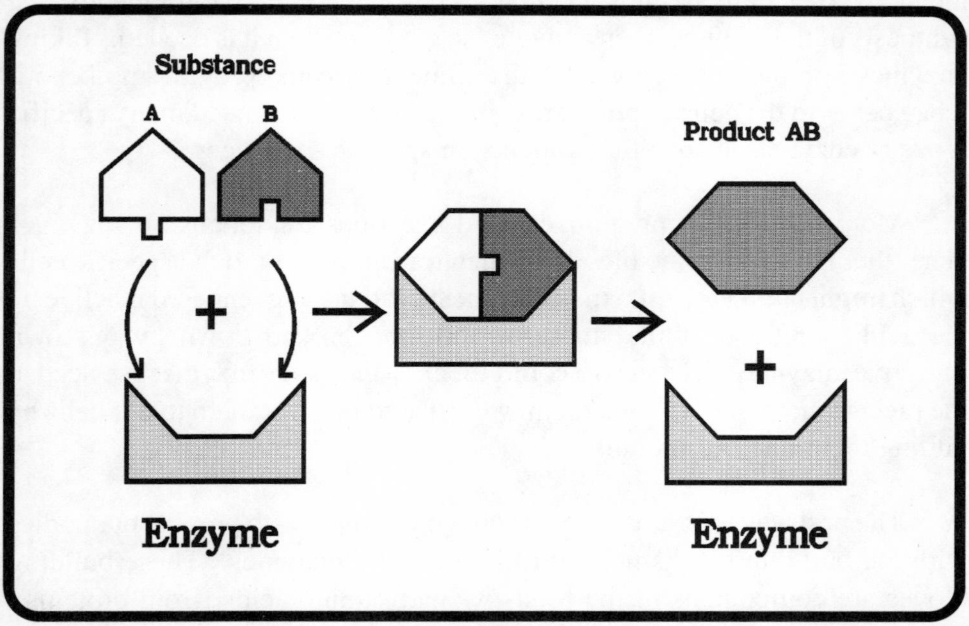

Hundreds of thousands of reactions are taking place in the cells of your body as you read this page. Your central nervous system is busy processing this information while your digestive system is processing your last meal. Your immune system is handling the many germs and particles which have entered your body, your heart is beating, and many cells are being made and replaced as other internal systems carry out a multitude of other intricate processes. **All** of these functions involve numerous enzymes.

Because enzymes are so important to everything our bodies do, some might think it a good idea to take enzyme pills and eat "enzyme-rich" foods. Unfortunately, with one very important exception, the enzymes in foods and pills have little to do with the enzymes needed in our bodies.

The countless enzymes in our bodies are **where** they are—in a specific place within a specific cell type, in a tissue, or in the blood—for very good and particular reasons. The environmental conditions of that specific area of the body (pH, temperature, chemical components, etc.) provide for the synthesis of the enzyme, then activate the enzyme when it is needed. Taking enzymes into the body by way of the alimentary canal provides no benefit whatsoever to the cells in other areas of the body, which need many specific types of enzymes at specific moments, in specific sequences.

More obviously, our stomachs and intestines cannot absorb enzymes, usher them intact into the blood and then transport them to the specific cells which might use them. Enzymes, like most proteins, are rendered inactive by the acid secretions of the stomach, and then broken down by our own digestive enzymes. Even if we **could** identify the exact enzymes we need at the precise moments we need them, we still couldn't get them to our cells by putting them into our mouths.

The best way to insure adequate enzyme activity is to provide our bodies with the building blocks needed to **make** those enzymes. These building blocks are components of the foods we eat: amino acids (from proteins), carbohydrates, vitamins, and minerals.

This brings us to the one enzyme exception we mentioned previously. The one type of enzyme which people **can** ingest to their benefit are the **digestive enzymes**. Three basic kinds of digestive enzymes break down the proteins, starches, and fats in the foods we eat. Normally our bodies do **make** these enzymes, but some individuals, due to disease, age, or stress, cannot manufacture adequate levels. As a result, these people cannot break down their foods sufficiently to provide nutrients in a form which can be absorbed.

Digestive enzymes are available in capsules. When ingested with foods, they may contribute to the digestion of those foods. It is possible for some of the **digestive** enzymes to survive the acid environment of the stomach. They need not be absorbed into the body to carry our their job in the small intestines. Few of the enzymes available in whole foods function as digestive enzymes.[7,57]

The foods we eat, like any life form, contain thousands of enzymes. Cereal grass is a virtual enzyme factory.[29] It contains proteases, amylases, and lipases—bustling with growth activity as it prepares itself for jointing.(See Chapter 1.) In the growing plant, countless specific enzymes are activated and deactivated at every moment, as chemical reactions spawn other chemical reactions according to growth stage, pH, temperature, etc. If they are not destroyed by processing, these enzymes can continue to function in the proper conditions even after the plant is harvested.

The level of potential enzyme activity retained in a plant after it is harvested depends on the way it is handled, stored, and packaged. Generally, protein (and therefore enzyme) structures are best retained when they are exposed to a minimum amount of light, air, and heat. When foods are stored for long periods in unfavorable conditions, or cooked in any way, their nutrient value is significantly reduced.

"**Live Foods**" is a term used in natural-food circles to refer to foods which are newly harvested and uncooked. Most people would agree that fresher is better, and they are right for many reasons. Fresher foods generally taste better, look better, smell better, and have higher levels of some nutrients than those long "separated from the vine".

Aside from all these visible and measurable advantages of "live foods", many health-conscious people feel that live foods provide an intangible, but important, benefit. This benefit is "**vitality**", or the quality of "**aliveness**" which live foods pass on to those who eat them. Some individuals say they can **see** and **feel** this quality in living systems, others have devices which they say help them to measure it. Most of us can't see or measure this vital energy, but would be hard pressed to deny its existence. Live foods may very well contain a kind of living energy which benefits us.

Many raw-food advocates incorrectly equate the benefits of this **vitality** with enzyme activity. Certainly, live foods contain active enzymes. But, as we have seen, enzymes are proteins which are digested and utilized by our body like any other proteins. **Ingested** enzymes do not generally provide our bodies with enhanced enzyme activity. If the quality of "**aliveness**" of foods is beneficial, it is for reasons other than the presence of enzymes which are still active in those foods **before** we eat them.

Enzymes and Live Foods: A Summary

Enzymes are proteins which stimulate vital chemical reactions in virtually every life process. All foods, when harvested, contain active enzymes. Foods which have been exposed to minimal levels of air, heat, and light may retain a high level of activatable enzymes.

Supplemental and food enzymes can potentially function in the digestive tract but have no direct effect on cells throughout the body.

Foods which are processed as little as possible are most desirable for nutrition, flavor, and aesthetic reasons. Fresh foods are also thought by many to provide an intangible benefit of **vitality**. If such a property exists, it cannot be attributed to any chemical enzyme activity which those foods convey to the cells of those who eat them.

Chapter 7

Green Foods for the Prevention of Diseases

> "There is absolutely no substitute for greens in the diet! If you refuse to eat these 'sunlight energy' foods you are depriving yourself, to a large degree, of the very essence of life."
>
> H. E. Kirschner, M.D.[63]

We have discussed the basic and essential functions of the individual nutrients contained in cereal grass and the other dark green vegetables. No one seriously believes, though, that the value of any food can be explained solely in terms of the individual nutrients contained in that food.

Nutrition studies tend to focus on the effects of isolated factors (vitamins, fatty acids, amino acids, etc.) on the growth or health state of test subjects or laboratory animals. Epidemiological nutrition studies, however, look for relationships between patterns of food consumption and the health status of entire populations. In the last decade, a large number of these types of studies have looked at health differences between people who eat green vegetables and those who don't. These studies have focused primarily on the relationships between cancer rates and the consumption of green vegetables.

Greens for the Intestines

As high fiber foods, dehydrated wheat and barley grasses are frequently taken for their positive effects on intestinal regularity. But the benefits provided by green vegetables to the digestive tract may extend to acute and chronic bowel diseases. The relationship of green food factors to the risk of colon cancer is discussed in Chapter 5.

A 1986 British medical study demonstrated that the consumption of all vegetables—particularly green vegetables—is significantly correlated with a reduction in the risk of appendicitis.[4]

Before World War II, Dr. Garnet Chaney at Stanford Medical School identified what he termed an **anti-peptic ulcer factor** in green vegetables and several other food materials.[20] Feeding five to ten grams of fresh greens or green vegetable juice daily to guinea pigs consistently protected them from the development of histamine-induced ulcers. No known nutrients could be substituted for this factor to produce comparable results.

Radiation Protection With Green Vegetables

Scientists have looked at the ability of green vegetables to protect animals from radiation damage since the 1930s (see Chapter 4). This type of research flourished in the 1950s and early 1960s, with the growing awareness of the dangers to humans posed by radiation.

In 1962, Doris Calloway and her colleagues gave lethal doses of X-radiation to healthy guinea pigs whose standard diet had been supplemented with a carefully controlled variety of foods and nutrients.[17] Ninety-seven per cent of the animals given no vegetable supplements died within twenty days. All of the vegetables containing beta-carotene provided some protection for the test animals. For example, only forty-four percent of the carrot-supplemented group died within twenty days. The dark green leafy vegetables provided, by far, the most protection from radiation. Only 12% of the animals fed mustard greens, and NONE of the animals fed alfalfa succumbed in 20 days.

It first appeared that beta-carotene could have been the protective factor in those experiments. However, when the stock diets of guinea pigs were supplemented with beta-carotene or vitamin A, little protection was provided. It seemed, then, that the radiation protection provided by the green vegetables was supplied by something other than the known nutrients. In their report, the investigators speculated that this radioprotective factor may parallel the water-soluble grass juice factor described earlier.

Green Vegetables and Cholesterol

Today, the use of several types of plant fiber (oat bran, apple pectin, psyllium seeds) is popular for the reduction of cholesterol. This practice is becoming widespread, though some authorities still question its benefits. A study of the impact of various whole vegetable foods on serum cholesterol was reported by Dr. Gary Fraser in the American Journal of Clinical Nutrition. In this study, all food supplements used had a positive effect, but "Calorie for calorie, the leafy vegetables seem to be most effective in lowering serum cholesterol."[38]

Animal experiments conducted in Japan indicate that the green juice of the cereal grass leaf has a cholesterol-lowering effect when given to rats with high cholesterol.[101]

Green Vegetables Against Cancer

Many studies have shown a higher than normal incidence of several kinds of cancer among populations consuming small quantities of green vegetables. These cancers are generally associated with the epithelial tissues that form the lining of many of our organs.

Lung cancer is the most lethal of all cancers for American men, and is rapidly becoming the leading killer of women as well. Many factors contribute to one's risk of getting lung cancer. The most potent risk factor is, of course, smoking. Anyone wishing to reduce the risk of getting this devastating disease should stop smoking now! Although no other single measure can improve one's prospects for a healthy future more directly, consumption of certain foods appears to affect one's risk of getting this disease. A large body of research indicates that eating dark green vegetables and foods high in beta-carotene may offer some protection from the development of lung cancer.[152]

One Italian study demonstrates that smokers who seldom eat green vegetables or carrots have several times the risk of getting lung cancer as smokers who consume green vegetables and carrots frequently. The investigators conclude that "Our data support a protective effect of vegetables. While it is possible that the nutrient responsible is carotene, the contribution of other substances present in the foods must be considered."[110]

Green vegetables may also be associated with a reduction in the risk of developing other types of cancer. A report in the Journal of the National Cancer Institute[46] indicates that hospital patients being treated for colon cancer have a history of eating fewer vegetables, especially green vegetables, than do other patients. Consumption of green vegetables has been shown to correlate with reduced risk of cancers of the ovary,[77] cervix,[139] and stomach.[78]

We have seen that green vegetables may offer some protection from the risk of epithelial cancers—those which affect the cells lining such organs as the lungs, colon, and ovaries. An interesting report in the American Journal of Clinical Nutrition[24] indicates that elderly people who eat the largest amount of green and yellow vegetables are the least likely to die of cancer of **all** types, whether or not they were smokers. The researchers state:

> "Our dietary data do indicate that, even in old age, higher intake of green and yellow vegetables is still associated with lowered risks of cancer deaths. It is still not known whether the protective relationship of such vegetables is truly one of cause and effect, and still less is known concerning which components of such vegetables are chiefly involved."

We can only echo the assertions made by these researchers. The information they provide suggests that eating green vegetables may indeed offer some protection from cancer.

It is unusual that so much research attention has focused on a specific type of food as a preventive agent for diseases. It is even more unique that these foods are distinguished by their color (dark green). We don't believe that this information would come as any surprise to our grandmothers.

PART THREE

FOOD CHOICES IN THE MODERN WORLD

"As the diseases of nutritional deficiency have diminished, they have been replaced by diseases of dietary excess and imbalance—problems that now rank among the leading causes of death in the United States, touch the lives of most Americans, and generate substantial health care costs."

—Surgeon General's Report
on Nutrition and Health,
July 27,1988[136]

By investing the time and effort required to read the foregoing seven chapters, you have, we hope, learned a good deal about green foods and why we need them. But for some the question still remains, "Why change? I've done all right so far with the foods I've been eating." The present section provides answers to this question.

The foods we eat may not be treating us as well as we think they are. Our ways of eating not only influence how we'll feel tomorrow, they might also help **determine** how we'll feel ten, twenty, or thirty years from now. Furthermore, the foods we consume as a society have a huge impact on our environment and natural resources. This, of course, also affects how we'll feel thirty years from now. There are plenty of reasons to pay attention to what we eat, and to make changes if necessary.

In this section we look first at the diets of our ancestors for clues about the kinds of foods for which our bodies may be best suited. We then look at the changes which have taken place in how we eat, in what we eat, and in our health status in relatively recent times.

Chapter 8

Is There a Diet Which Is "NATURAL" For Humans?

Our diets aren't what they used to be, but our bodies are. Scientists say our species (**Homo sapiens**) has been here for about 40,000 years, and that we really have not physically changed much in that time. Human-like primates have been here for about four million years. Yet we have cultivated our food—crops and livestock—for only about 10,000 years. Before that time, our ancestors ate what they could forage or hunt. In some parts of the world, the diets of traditional and tribal peoples still resemble those of our ancestors. The diseases which plague these people are very different from the ailments faced by those in the more "developed" countries.

Today, humans are faced with health problems which were previously of minor importance. Because these diseases occur primarily in people of post-reproductive ages, we inherit little resistance to them. Our immune arsenal is not designed to cope with industrialized 20th century diseases nor, perhaps, with some of the dietary practices we indulge in today.

Many physicians and nutritionists feel that Western dietary practices which have developed over the last fifty to a hundred years are responsible for the prevalence of the most deadly diseases we face today.[31] Heart and artery diseases, some cancers, and diabetes are sometimes called **The**

Diseases of Civilization. They are responsible for most deaths in the industrial countries of the world. They are troubling not only because they are so common, and take such a heavy toll, but because we generally have no effective treatments against them. The best hope we have of reducing the incidence of heart disease and cancer is to **prevent** them.

These diseases are quite rare in traditional, non-Western cultures and were rare among our ancestors as well. They are also extremely rare in the other primates. The differences between our lives and theirs is not limited, of course, to the foods we eat. Health and disease differences result from dietary, environmental, work pattern, psycho-social, and other lifestyle/ cultural elements. But a large body of evidence suggests that dietary differences are a major reason why we get the Diseases of Civilization and they do not.

The last hundred years has brought a completely new way of living and eating to our part of the world. Although refined sugars and flours were eaten before that time, the per capita consumption of these foods has multiplied many times over in recent decades. The increased use of breaded and fried convenience foods, grain-fed and fattened antibiotic-laden beef, pork and poultry, flavor enhancers, food colorings and preservatives has been accompanied by a drastic reduction in the consumption of unadulterated fruits and vegetables. Although we are living to older ages, many of those older years are often spent in poor health.

We may well wonder, then, if there is a way of eating which our bodies were "designed" to handle—a way of eating which we can adopt to prevent the occurrence of these Diseases of Civilization.

What Did Our Ancestors Eat?

The hunting/gathering diet consumed by all people on earth until the development of agriculture was refined over many thousands, perhaps millions, of years.[32] The human gastro-intestinal tract adapted to this type of diet over the same time span. Of course, the specific foods used varied from era to era and from area to area, but research suggests that the same **kinds** of foods were consistently used in the different populations of early humans.

Vegetarians and carnivores both like to think that their way of eating is most "natural", claiming that ancestral diets consisted mainly of plant foods or wild animals, respectively. But the archaeological evidence suggests that evolving humans went through a number of dietary phases which included less, then more, then less reliance on animal foods. The human digestive system has the capacity to obtain nutrients from a wide variety of food types.[52]

The pre-hominids of the Miocene era (25 million years ago) are thought to have eaten a fruit-based diet.[32] Hominids emerged between 4.5 and 7.5 million years ago, with diets including slightly more meat, either from scavenging or hunting. As our ancestors became more adept at tool use, meat became more important in their diet.[31] Many tools were developed for processing game. These hominids often lived in areas where they had access to herds of grazing animals. **Homo erectus** and early **Homo sapiens** are thought to have had diets containing about half plant foods and half animal foods.[31]

Our Stone Age ancestors had to cope with "lean periods" of food scarcity. Researchers have speculated that early hominids developed a taste for foods which have high fat or sugar contents.[32,52] These foods provided a concentrated source of calories, allowing the short-term storage of fat reserves to see our active ancestors through those lean times. The "sweet tooths" and "fat tooths", which served our ancestors in times of need, contribute to widespread obesity and consumption of calorie rich/nutrient lean foods in modern Western societies where food is abundantly available.

The use of animal foods again declined before the inception of agriculture. Food consumption shifted to a subsistence pattern, with tools being developed for the gathering and processing of wild plant foods. Hunter/gatherer cultures in existence today have a diet very much like that of these ancestors.

The development of agriculture, about 10,000 years ago, brought dramatic changes to the human diet and way of life.[137] Population centers stabilized. Meat use declined dramatically, with plant foods comprising as much as ninety percent of the human diet.[31]

With the advent of agriculture, grains and cereals became the staple foods of our ancestors, as they continue to be for most of the world's population. Vegetable protein foods (beans, seeds and grains) replaced animal protein foods. Humans no longer had to depend on seasonal plant foods and roaming herds as their food sources. They stayed in one place and often gathered in large communities. The stage was set for the development of the ancient civilizations from which we trace our cultural roots.

The meat consumed by ancient people was wild game. That meat was considerably lower in fat than the "bred" meats we eat today. Wild game meat typically contains three to five percent fat, while meat from modern cattle can contain up to 30% fat.[31] Also, the fat in wild game is quite different from that of domestic livestock animals. The wild game meats consumed by our ancestors were considerably higher in protein and lower in fat than the meat consumed today. Of course, wild game contained none of the antibiotics, hormones or other "medicines" found in our modern livestock animals.

Our ancestors consumed complex carbohydrates, as opposed to the simple sugars eaten in large quantities today. If any alcoholic beverages were consumed, they were fermented, not distilled, and so had lower levels of alcohol than is contained in our modern spirits.

The foods consumed by these hunter/gathering people were extremely high in the nutrients (vitamins, minerals, proteins) that we now consider essential for good health. Potassium intake was greater than sodium intake. Today, in most parts of the world, the reverse is true.[32] These diets also contained a significantly lower level of saturated fats than is found in modern diets. It is now generally accepted that high consumption of fats, particularly saturated fats, contributes to the heart and artery diseases which are the most debilitating and deadly to Western populations.

It is also thought that our ancestors retained a relatively high level of physical fitness throughout their lives. Skeletal remains indicate that they retained a high degree of muscular strength into old age, considerably higher than that of a modern Westerner.[32]

Some information about dietary adaptations may also be derived from studying the diets of our closest "relatives" in the animal kingdom, the great apes (gorillas and chimpanzees). The diet of the great apes is almost exclusively plant matter, particularly wild green vegetation. These foods contain very large quantities of chlorophyll, beta-carotene, vegetable protein, and, of course, fiber. The large intestines of the great apes is longer than that of humans, and so is better adapted to the digestion of huge quantities of cellulose fibers.

Both humans and apes are well suited to the digestion of hemi-cellulose fibers.[92] It is thought by some archaeologists that the shorter colon of humans allows them to consume smaller quantities of more concentrated foods while maintaining a relatively large body size, compared to the apes who consume large quantities of lower caloric foods. This adaptation is skewed when humans consume large quantities of high-calorie, high-fat, low-fiber foods. Besides the obvious hazards associated with these foods, they tend to provide a very limited variety of vitamins and minerals.

The Ancestral Diet in the Twentieth Century

More than fifty twentieth century hunter/gatherer societies have been studied by anthropologists. The diets of these people are thought to resemble those consumed by our ancestors, and so might be considered an approximation of the kinds of foods our bodies are best adapted to.

The Kadi San Bushmen of the Kalahari are perhaps the best studied of the modern hunter/gatherers.[137] Their diet is somewhat similar to that of some non-human omnivores. Some may find it surprising that so little animal prey is consumed by these people, who subsist mainly on foraged foods.

Modern hunter/gatherers, with the exception of those in Arctic areas, typically consume a diet consisting of 65% vegetation and 35% animal foods. Approximately 20% of their daily calories come from fat. (In Western countries, diets typically derive 40-45% of their calories from fat.) Their diets are also low in salt and refined sugars and include a wide variety of complex carbohydrates, high intake of fiber and moderate calorie consumption.

With respect to the diseases which plague **us** most, these people are considerably better off than we are. They tend to have stable blood pressures into old age. Few of them are obese; heart attacks, strokes and diabetes are relatively rare. The cancers most common in our culture—cancers of the lungs, colon, breast, and prostate, are virtually non-existent among modern hunter/gatherers.

It cannot be said, however, that those who live a more traditional, hunter/gatherer lifestyle generally enjoy better health than those of us in the West. The infectious diseases, which are much less lethal to us, are still rampant in these "developing" parts of the world. This is due to inferior sanitation and water purification practices, as well as the poor availability of medicines which counteract bacterial and parasitic infections. As a result, these people frequently have diseases rarely encountered in "developed" areas of the world.

The relatively low incidence of degenerative diseases in developing countries is not due only to the fact that individuals in these countries have a shorter life expectancy. The diseases of civilization described earlier are rarely seen, even among the old people, in these areas. In addition, the younger people in non-industrialized areas do not exhibit the early symptoms and tendencies towards those diseases commonly seen in the young people of Western nations.[31]

A large number of studies of traditional African diets suggest that minerals, vitamins and proteins, previously thought to be best obtained from meat and dairy products, **can** be absorbed in sufficient quantities from nutrient-rich vegetation. It has long been known that the many species of wild green plants consumed in rural regions of Africa are, for those populations, important sources of protein, calcium, vitamin A, vitamin C and iron.[36]

In the Usambara Mountain region of northern Tanzania, the staple food consumed at almost every meal is a stiff porridge made from maize meal or another starchy vegetable. In addition, most meals contain at least one side dish, the most common of which is some type of michicha, one of the over 40 wild green plants growing in the area.[36]

Nutritional wisdom can be found both in modern scientific texts, and in observation of the practices of people who have successfully developed their ways of living and eating over thousands of years. Unfortunately, in many parts of the world, traditional food consumption patterns are being abandoned in favor of the "quick-fix" sweetened, fattened foods of the modern Western nations. As traditional diets and ways of life become more "modernized", the pattern of the Diseases of Civilization in developing nations is shifting to resemble those of industrialized societies.

Is our convenient, processed food supply out of step with our Stone Age physiology? Should we attempt to maintain a diet more like that consumed when our digestive system was still in the formative stages? The truth is that the actual foods regularly eaten by our hunter/gatherer ancestors are not readily available to us today. They ate **wild** plants and **wild** animals, which are quite distinct from our domesticated food sources. The stress demands and survival pressures put upon us by our modern world and environment are different from those experienced by our ancestors. For ecological, aesthetic, and practical reasons, it would be undesirable to try to go back to those dietary ways of old.

But we can take steps to emulate the **types** of foods and nutrients consumed by early humans. Features of the dietary patterns of our hunter/gatherer ancestors are summarized below:

-A wide variety of complex carbohydrates from fruits, wild greens, tubers, and roots were consumed.

-The ratio of animal to plant foods varied from 50/50 to 10/90 animal/plant foods.

-Meats, when eaten, were extremely low in fat.

-Calorie consumption was in proportion to expenditure.

The characteristics of this food consumption pattern demonstrate that the diet of our ancestors had some similarities to the dietary recommendations made by the American Heart Association, The U.S. Surgeon General, and most national and world agencies which make dietary recommendations. Adopting a diet which more closely resembles that of our ancestors may provide health benefits to modern people living in our faster-paced, post-industrial society.

Chapter 9

Health Hazards of the Modern Diet

> "Next in importance to the divine profusion of water, light and air . . . may be reckoned the universal beneficence of grass. It yields no fruit in Earth or air, yet should its harvest fail for a single year famine would depopulate the world."
>
> Senator John James Ingalls, 1872.

The closing years of the twentieth century present many challenges to the modern inhabitant of the planet Earth. Certain health concerns and problems are in many ways unique to people living in our time. Changes in social structures, ways of living and working, the natural environment, and available foods and medicines all combine to provide living conditions quite different from those in which our ancestors lived.

Some segments of our society are becoming more conscious of fitness and health. Many are making positive changes in their diets. As the life span of the individual continues to increase, the common perception is that we are healthier than ever before. All of these facts sound encouraging, but let's take a closer look.

The following information is taken from the U.S. Surgeon General's Report on Nutrition and Health, released to the public on July 27, 1988.[136]

Our hearts and arteries aren't doing too well. Fifty-eight million Americans have high blood pressure, including 39 million who are under age 65. About 1.5 million people have heart attacks each year in the United States. One third of them don't survive. Half a million Americans have strokes each year.

The second leading cause of death in the U.S. (after cardiovascular diseases) is cancer. Most of us are related to or know someone who has experienced this dread disease. Every year, about a million new cases are reported, with almost half a million people dying from cancer each year.

About eleven million Americans are said to have diabetes, but almost half of them have not been diagnosed. This disease can kill, either directly or through its many complications.

Approximately 34 million adults in the U.S. are obese. Social and fashion considerations aside, obesity puts one at greater risk for heart disease, high blood pressure, diabetes, some types of cancer and other chronic diseases.

The Surgeon General also reports that up to seventy percent of people between the ages of forty and seventy are affected with some form of diverticular disease, or problems with the intestines. Most of these cases are undiagnosed.

Fifteen to twenty million Americans are affected to some extent by osteoporosis, or "porous bones". This condition is associated with easily fractured vertebrae and other bones.

What these diseases have in common is that they are all considered age-related conditions, or "degenerative diseases". They have also been called "The Diseases of Civilization", as described in the previous chapter. Heart disease, cancer, and diabetes are responsible for the majority of deaths in the United States. While more of us are living to an older age, most of us are not enjoying good health for many of our later years.

Medical science has provided us with many spectacular health benefits. Perhaps the most striking breakthroughs in modern medicine occurred in the 1940s and 1950s with the development of antibiotics and several important vaccines. These "miracle" medicines have dramatically reduced the incidence of infectious diseases in Western countries. Infant mortality has diminished; many more children now survive into adulthood. Infectious diseases which previously posed serious health risks for people of all ages are now treatable and have, in some cases, been nearly eradicated.

Some progress has been made in the detection and diagnosis of the degenerative diseases which are now the most serious threats to our health. A number of treatments are used (surgery, chemotherapy, painkillers, radiation) to interfere with the progression of these diseases, or to treat their symptoms. These treatments are generally not considered cures. The long term prognosis for people suffering from cancer or heart disease is often poor.

In spite of massive governmental and private effort and investment, we still have no cures for the diseases which plague us most. This is not particularly surprising, given the nature of these illnesses.

An infectious disease is the direct consequence of the uncontrolled growth of germs. There may be a multitude of reasons why those germs are able to grow in the specific tissues they infect, but by limiting the growth of the germs, the infection and the disease it causes can be controlled.

The degenerative diseases are different. They are caused by many factors. Immunity, heredity, infections, environment, lifestyle, and psychological factors are all thought to interact to determine an individual's probability of getting cancer. Many of the same factors have been identified as instrumental in the cause and prevention of heart disease. Because there are **no single causes for the chronic degenerative diseases**, it is not surprising that **no simple medical cures** have been found.

This picture, from the traditional point of view, looks rather bleak. But a closer look at the factors which cause these diseases provides a more optimistic view. Except for heredity, all of these disease-causing factors can be altered through the individual's own efforts. These diseases are largely preventable! If this seems unbelievable, consider the following. The incidence of lung cancer, the most deadly of all cancers in this country, is quite low among non-smokers, and even lower among non-smokers living outside of large city areas. There are other risk factors for this disease, such as hazardous occupations and low intake of green vegetables. The incidence of heart disease is frequently associated with diet, exercise, work habits, and psychological variables, all of which can be changed to one's health advantage!

Change is not easy for most of us. We would, perhaps, like to know which specific things we can do to improve our health outlook without radically altering our way of life. For instance, many of us would not be willing to change occupations or places of residence unless we had dramatic proof that our health status would be directly impacted. As stated in the Surgeon General's Report:

> "For the two out of three adult Americans who do not smoke and do not drink excessively, one personal choice seems to influence long-term health prospects more than any other: What we eat. . . .

> "What we eat may affect our risk for several of the leading causes of death for Americans, notably, coronary heart disease, stroke, atherosclerosis, diabetes, and some types of cancer. These disorders now account for more than two-thirds of all deaths in the United States."[136]

Given the wide array of degenerative diseases, one might wonder whether enough dietary changes could be made to have a significant effect on our health. Indeed, many people now feel that almost everything they eat and do is said to be hazardous to their health. But there really is good news: The dietary changes which can minimize our risk of chronic diseases are remarkably similar! In other words, the same basic dietary habits may help protect us from several, and possibly most, of the common degenerative diseases.

There is a general consistency in the dietary recommendations made by various scientific, governmental, and private health agencies. Although there is a great deal to know about nutrition and its relationship to disease, the suggestions made by these groups are relatively simple. They rely heavily on moderation and common sense. Most people are already aware of these recommendations:

-Reduce consumption of fats and cholesterol.

-Increase consumption of vegetables, fruits, and whole grain foods.

-Reduce consumption of refined, simple sugars; increase intake of complex carbohydrates.

-Reduce sodium intake.

-Consume alcohol only in moderation, if at all.

-Achieve and maintain proper body weight.

All of this seems pretty simple. Different agencies include slight variations on more specific recommendations, such as six vs. four daily servings of fruits and vegetables. Each agency recommends including **at least** one serving of a dark green or orange vegetable every day.[15]

The general consensus is for an increased intake of plant foods—whole grains, fruits, vegetables, and legumes, with their abundance of vitamins, minerals, complex carbohydrates and fiber. This is to be accompanied by a reduced reliance on high-fat, no-fiber animal foods, with their high levels of cholesterol and calories.

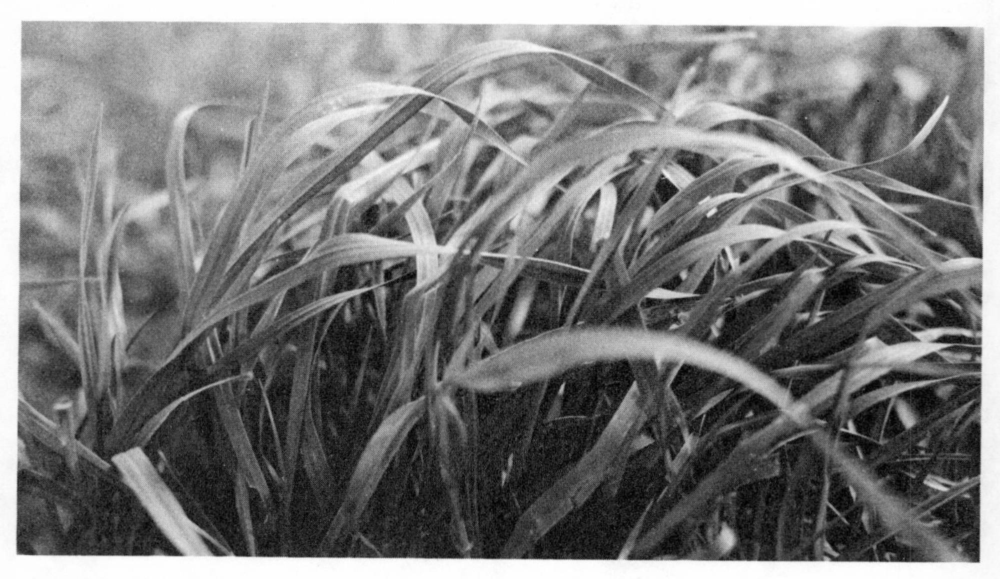

Nutrition research can now tell us **why** green foods are important in our diet, and can also identify the specific health benefits which they provide. Dehydrated cereal grass is an excellent and convenient source of these nutritional benefits. Simply increasing the amount of dark green vegetable foods would be a significant upgrade of what is considered the "average" American diet.

The kinds of foods we eat are not the only source of health hazards associated with our diet. Diseases caused by food toxins have been identified throughout history. Some substances which occur naturally in foods can cause us problems. Alkaloids are present in commonly consumed foods and herbs, as are a variety of enzyme inhibitors. Substances such as oxalates and phytates inhibit the absorption of required nutrients. These substances are generally not consumed in quantities sufficient to cause noticeable health problems.

Only in the present century have we been exposed to toxins which are **intentionally** added to crops and processed foods. Food additives have been around for several decades now, and evaluations of the safety or hazards of their long term use can now be made. Estimates of the hazards of newer food additives rely largely on animal experiments. But about three dozen of the pesticides currently in use have not even been tested for their cancer-causing potential.[87]

The list of toxic chemicals we are exposed to in foods is extremely long. Residues from fertilizers and pesticides are common in fresh and processed foods. A wide variety of preservatives, colorings, and flavor enhancers are present in packaged and prepared foods. These convenient, prepared, beautifully colored and flavor-enhanced foods are often most compatible with our lifestyles and taste preferences. Our food choices are no longer limited by local availability of foods in season, or by rapid spoilage of those foods once they are processed. But, as is always the case, there is a high price to pay for these luxuries.

According to a report released by the National Academy of Science in May, 1987, fifteen of the most commonly consumed American foods contain pesticide residues that constitute nearly 80 percent of the estimated dietary cancer risk for humans.[138] The scientists writing the report concluded that discrepancies in standards enforced by federal agencies permit more carcinogens in our foods than the law intends. They state that "the rules must be updated and made consistent if the public health is to be effectively protected." Environmentalists claim that these estimates are actually low, because they do not consider the many carcinogens contained in our air and water supplies, which interact with and add to the hazards posed by food contaminants.[146]

Over 390,000 TONS of pesticides are used each year in the United States alone. That's over 3 pounds for each person.[87] Ninety percent of all fungicides, 60% of all herbicides and 30% of all insecticides have been shown to cause cancer in animals.[138] The greatest risk, according to the NAS report, comes from pesticide residues found on tomatoes. Next on the list is beef, then potatoes. The remaining most common foods, in order of estimated hazard, are oranges, lettuce, apples, peaches, pork, wheat, soybeans, beans, carrots, chicken, corn, and grapes.

Remember, these are cancer hazards posed only by pesticide residues. This does not take into account the large number of steroid hormones, antibiotics, and ingested contaminants associated with livestock production. Organic produce is not available to most of us. Consumer groups advocate washing conventionally-grown produce with soapy water before eating it. There is not much that can be done about chemical contamination of animal products. Wheat grass and other cereal grasses can be produced without chemical sprays because they are harvested in the early spring before pesticides are "needed."

Modern farming and food production methods put more than our personal health at risk. Dr. Michael Fox, an environmental activist, calls our industrialized approach to farming agricide, or "the failure of the agricultural food production system to be sustainable—ecologically, economically, and in terms of contributing positively to our health".[141]

Intensive fertilization, plowing, and single-crop farming depletes soil nutrients and the volume of topsoils. Agrichemicals now pollute our aquifers, the underground lakes which supply water to many communities. Topsoil, the rich, relatively loose earth which supplies the nutrient and growth medium for our food crops, is being depleted at a rapid rate. This resource builds up over many centuries, and is not quickly replaceable. Agribusinesses are run for maximum short term productivity and profit, with little concern for the effects of farming techniques on the health of the soils or the nutrients contained in the foods.

The availability and distribution of food in the world today is as ironic as it is troubling. While billions of people throughout the world struggle to feed themselves, large numbers of Americans and Europeans struggle to avoid **over**feeding themselves. A further irony is that many of the overfat, over-caloried people in the affluent world are themselves poorly nourished. The effective and equitable supply of adequate food to people around the world will require a mixture of goodwill, economic maneuvering and political expertise. The most important ingredient, perhaps, is the interest and will to effect such changes.

The food preferences of Western affluent nations affect much more than the coronary arteries of the people living in these countries. Although there is currently sufficient grain to feed all people in all nations of the world, our overwhelming preference for meat-centered meals is a drain on the world's resources.[52,84]

The destruction of millions of acres of tropical rain forest in Central and South America continues in order to provide range land for beef cattle. Who buys that beef? Primarily, American fast food hamburger chain customers.[52] The destruction of the rain forests dooms countless species of plants and animals, and dramatically increases the level of carbon dioxide in our atmosphere.

The point here is not to alarm those who are already aware of these issues. The point, rather, is to underline the fact that our food choices have long range effects on our health. We who can make choices about the foods we eat must be aware that our choices have an effect on **more** than our own bodies; these choices ultimately affect the health of our planet and all of its inhabitants.

The many hazards associated with modern foods and "civilized" diets may seem to be too great a problem to overcome. But that pessimistic notion really misses the point we are making. The diseases most prevalent in our modern culture are largely **preventable** by choices we can make concerning our own diets and lifestyles. And in the big picture, the changes which can improve our own personal health prospects are compatible with dietary patterns which are the most sound ecologically.

Observations and Conclusions

"There is a mysterious something about the grasses—a power, a spirit, a mystique—that both stirs the soul and quiets it. 'Sometimes I feel the whole world's flying to pieces', one farmer says. 'Then I take my dog and go out in my beautiful grass, and I know it isn't so.'"

—James and Alice Wilson[149]

Chapter 10

The Forest, The Trees, and The Leaves

"Health is beauty, and the most perfect health is the most perfect beauty."

—William Shemstone (1714-1763)

The color green is associated with plant life, and symbolically with vitality and healing. In the previous pages we have seen some of the ways in which eating green foods can improve and sustain our health, and why the cereal grasses are superior green vegetables. It is important now to step out from among the trees of individual nutrient functions, to look at the forest—the big picture of good health and how it may fit into the picture of a good life. Ultimately, the measure of a healthy life is the extent to which we feel good in our bodies, in our relationships, in our communities, and in the world at large.

We are in a position to emphasize the important influence of diet on good health; that is the area we are most informed about. We think a part of being healthy is dietary awareness, but know that it is only a part.

The simple fact is, the types of foods which offer us the most protection from long term diseases are similar to the ones consumed by our ancestors. There seems to be every reason to get with it, dietarily speaking. But most folks are hesitant to make big changes in how they eat, even if they can see the clear advantages for themselves, for their families, and for the health of the planet.

We in the technologically developed countries can no longer afford the luxury of eating only the foods which taste best to us. Our modern taste preferences are conditioned to favor foods which are unbalanced in the direction of sweetness, saltiness, and fat content. It no longer makes sense to keep putting into your mouth whatever food is available and convenient and expect that it will all work out somehow.

Alot of information about health and diet is being circulated these days. Perhaps a specialist could sort through all of this information, but most of us need some kind of an overview of what makes us healthy and what makes us sick. Then with a little common sense and a few basic nutritional facts we can make our own informed choices about our diet and health practices.

> "As long as a person takes active exercise, works hard, does not overeat, and keeps his bowels open, he will be free, even though the food he eats be coarse."
>
> --Moses Miamonides (1135-1204 A.D.)

According to some of the nature-cure advocates of the early 20th century, maintaining good health is really not complicated at all! They claimed that good health depends, simply, on the maintenance of proper assimilations and proper eliminations. This means providing our bodies with adequate nutrients and the wherewithal to get rid of the waste products of metabolism, cell debris and disease-causing elements. The body, given the proper tools and relieved of an excessive burden of backed up waste products, can achieve a state of health which far surpasses anything a doctor can provide for us with medicines. The combination of nutrient absorbtion and healthy bowel function provides a base on which abundant health is built.

This health overview still makes a lot of sense. The oldest health insurance is vis medicatrix naturae, or the healing power of nature described by Hippocrates. The best and most lasting cures are those which allow the body to heal itself, for no medical treatment can possibly cover all the physiological bases without jamming up a few of them. We need nutritionally adequate food, air, and sunshine in order to thrive, and in order for our self-healing mechanisms to operate.

The really good foods provide valuable substances for both assimilation and elimination. The most beneficial vitamin and mineral foods are roughage-containing plant foods which are deeply colored, such as the dark green and orange vegetables, and many of the fruits. Starchy foods such as whole grains and potatoes, which contain complex carbohydrates, are the best sources of food energy. They are often also excellent fiber foods. Proteins are most concentrated in animal foods, but are abundant also in fiber-containing beans, seeds, nuts, whole grains, and cereal grasses.

From this perspective, the ideal diet would include a wide variety of plant foods. Animal foods would be included, if at all, as supplemental foods. This would allow the intake and absorption of all of the vital nutrients which our bodies need. It would also minimize the fatty foods and toxic breakdown products which our bodies need to eliminate. In addition, an abundance of unrefined plant foods in the diet provides ample amounts of all the food fibers which enhance proper elimination of waste products.

This simple approach to food consumption also describes the basic diet consumed in those areas of the world which are not plagued by heart diseases and many of the cancers common in our society.

It's really not that difficult to change what you eat! The hard part is facing whatever it is that makes you think you couldn't possibly change something so basic. Even if your palate is trained to like cheeseburgers and chocolate milkshakes, believe us—it is possible that you may one day like vegetable casseroles just as much, and that you might even come to find the burger and milkshake extremely distasteful. Most of us are former burger lovers.

Personal change is really only possible when you **want** to change. You probably really **do** want to feel better physically and better about your place in the world. The two most important tools you'll need are information and patience with yourself. As far as information goes, don't believe everything you hear or read. Get some basic information, then test out the particulars on yourself to see which ones apply to you.

The Bigger Picture

It takes more than a change of diet to get healthy and make the world a better place. Diet is only one important factor involved in our health. The other obvious contributors are exercise, adequate rest, fresh air, and moderate exposure to sunlight. The less obvious requirements for good health are involvement in satisfying social and personal relationships, and in work which is interesting and fulfilling.

Those of us who have worked extensively with information related to the well-being of the physical body are aware that such a state involves the assimilation of a wide spectrum of nourishing elements. We are nourished not only by foods and oxygen, but by giving and receiving love and inspiration, and by facing challenges and experiencing personal growth. If any of these processes is trivialized or ignored, we can never be really healthy.

Your good health and fulfilling life are important not only to you and to your family, they are important to all the rest of us as well. Please nourish yourself to the best of your ability. Maintaining an adequate level of green foods in your diet will contribute in many ways to your physical health.

But "eating more green" can mean much more than consuming your daily quota of green vegetables. Green is the color of life and growth on this Earth. Many of us are moving through our daily routines unaware of the vibrancy and joy of living which is abundantly available to every one of us. Green plants not only feed us, they provide us with the oxygen which is our breath of life, and with an example of the beauty of the changes that come with the seasons—the undaunted life energy that bursts forth in a mighty green blast every spring, no matter how harsh the winter which has passed.

We encourage you to take the steps in your life which you know will contribute to your health. If you are currently thriving, we thank you for the example and inspiration which you are providing for the rest of us. If your health and joy of life are not at full potential, **"Eat more green!"**. It's all around you.

References

1. Anderson, J. 1986. Fiber and health: an overview. American Journal of Gastroenterology 10:892-897.

2. Anderson, J. 1983. Plant fiber and blood pressure. Annals of Internal Medicine 98:842-846.

3. Baker, H. 1978. Plants and Civilization. Wadsworth Publishing Co. Belmont, CA.

4. Barker, D., Morris, J., and Nelson, M. 1986. Vegetable consumption and acute appendicitis in 59 areas in England and Wales. British Medical Journal of Clinical Research Education 292:927-30.

5. Battersby, A. 1988. Biosynthesis of the pigments of life. Journal of Natural Products 51:629-42.

6. Baxter, J. and Steinberg, D. 1967. Absorption of phytol from dietary chlorophyll in the rat. Journal of Lipid Research 8:615-620.

7. Beck, C. and Scott, D. 1974. Enzymes in foods—for better or worse. in: Food Related Enzymes. J. Whitaker, Ed. American Chemical Society. Washington, D.C.

8. Bendich, A. and Shapiro, S. 1986. Effect of beta-carotene and canthaxamin on the immune responses of the rat. Journal of Nutrition 116:2254-2262.

9. Berg, J. 1975. Can nutrition explain the pattern of international epidemiology of hormone-dependent cancers? Cancer Research 35:3345-3350.

10. Bing, F., Secretary, AMA Council on Foods. 1939. Accepted Foods—Cerophyll. The Journal of the American Medical Association 112:733.

11. Borasky, R. and Bradbury, J. 1942. Frozen plant juice as the source of a rabbit ovulating factor. American Journal of Physiology 137:637-639.

12. Bradbury, J. 1944. The rabbit ovulating factor of plant juice. American Journal of Physiology 142:487-493.

13. Bronowski, Jacob. 1973. The Ascent of Man. Little, Brown, & Company, Boston and Toronto.

14. Buffalo Courier Express June 1, 1942. "Fed His Family Grass for Eleven Years".

15. Butrum, R. Clifford, C. and Lanza, E. 1988. NCI dietary guidelines: rationale. American Journal of Clinical Nutrition 48:888-895.

16. Caldwell, J. and Jakoby, W., Eds. 1983. Biological Basis of Detoxification. Academic Press. New York.

17. Calloway, D., Newell, G., Calhoun, W. and Munson, A. 1962. Further studies of the influence of diet on radiosensitivity of guinea pigs, with special reference to broccoli and alfalfa. Journal of Nutrition 79:340-348.

18. Cannon. M. and Emerson, G. 1939. Dietary requirements of the guinea pig with reference to the need for a special factor. The Journal of Nutrition 18:155-167.

19. Carpenter, E. 1949. Clinical experiences with chlorophyll preparations with a particular reference to chronic osteomyelitis and chronic ulcers. American Journal of Surgery. Feb.1949.

20. Cheney, G. 1950. Anti-peptic ulcer dietary factor. Journal of the American Dietetic Association 26:668-672.

21. Chernomorsky, S., and Segelman, A. 1988. Biological activities of chlorophyll derivatives. New Jersey Medicine 85:669-673.

22. Clasen, A. 1939. Hypovitaminosis and its relationship to disease. Kansas City Medical Journal May, 1939, p. 23.

23. Clydesdale, F. and Francis, F. 1985. Food Nutrition and Health. AVI Publishing Co. Westport.

24. Colditz, G., Branch, L., Lipnick, R., Willett, W., Rosner, B., Posner, B., and Hennekens, C. 1985. Increased green and yellow vegetable intake and lowered cancer deaths in an elderly population. The American Journal of Clinical Nutrition 41:32-36.

25. Colio, L. and Babb, V. 1948. Study of a new stimulatory growth factor. Journal of Biological Chemistry 174:405-409.

26. Collings, G. 1945. Chlorophyll and adrenal cortical extract in the local treatment of burns. American Journal of Surgery 70:58-63.

27. Cunha, T. Ross, O., Phillips, P. and Bohstedt, G. 1944. Further observations on the dietary insufficiency of a corn-soybean ration for reproduction of swine. Journal of Animal Science 3:415.

28. Devadas, R. and Murthy, N. 1978. Biological utilization of B-carotene from amaranth and leaf protein in preschool children. World Review of Nutrition and Diet 31:159-161.

29. Duffus, C.M. and Duffus, J.H. 1984. Carbohydrate Metabolism in Plants. Longman. London and New York.

30. Eastwood, M. 1987. Dietary fiber and the risk of cancer. Nutrition Reviews 45:193-197.

31. Eaton, S. and Konner, M. 1985. Paleolithic nutrition — a consideration of its nature and current implications. New England Journal of Medicine 5:283-289.

32. Eaton, S. and Shostak, M. 1986. Fat tooth blues. Natural History 7:6-12.

33. Erschoff, B. 1957. Beneficial effects of alfalfa and other succulent plants on the growth of immature guinea pigs fed a mineralized dried milk ration. Journal of Nutrition 62:295-312.

34. Erschoff, B. and Hernandez, H. 1960. An unidentified water-soluble factor in alfalfa which improves utilization of vitamin A. Journal of Nutrition 70:313-320.

35. Fisher, H. Scott, H. and Hansen, R. 1954. Further studies on the alfalfa factor and its relation to the liver and whey factors. Journal of Nutrition 52:13-24.

36. Fleuret, A. 1979. The role of wild foliage plants in the diet; a case study from Lushoto, Tanzania. Ecology of Food and Nutrition 8:87-93.

37. Fox, P. and Condon, J., Eds. 1982. Food Proteins. Applied Science Publishers. London and New York.

38. Fraser, G., Jacobs, D., Anderson, J., Foster, N., Palta, M. and Blackburn, H. 1981. The effect of various vegetable supplements on serum cholesterol. American Journal of Clinical Nutrition 34:1272-1277.

39. Friedman, M. and Mitchell, J. 1941. Variations in the yield of gonadotropic material from green plants in relation to the season of growth and the pH of the fresh juice. Endocrinology 29:172-178.

40. Gallagher, J., Biscoe, P., and Wallace, J. 1979. Field studies of cereal leaf growth. Journal of Experimental Botany 30:657-668.

41. Gardner, F., Pearce, R., and Mitchell, R. 1985. Photosynthesis. In Physiology of Plant Crops. Iowa State University Press. Ames, Iowa.

42. Gershwin, M., Beach, R., Hurley, L. 1985. Nutrition and Immunity. Academic Press. Orlando.

43. Golden, T. 1956. Effective management of offensive odors. Gastroenterology 31:260.

44. Gordon, B. 1942. Grass goes on the diet list. The Sunday Star, Washington D.C., October 18, 1942.

45. Gould, F.W. 1968. Grass Systematics. McGraw-Hill. New York.

46. Graham, S., Dayal, H., Swanson, M., Mittelman, A., and Wilkinson, G. 1978. Diet in the epidemiology of cancer of the colon and rectum. Journal of the National Cancer Institute. 61:709-714.

47. Graham, W., Kohler, G. and Schnabel, C. 1940. "Grass As A Food: Vitamin Content". Paper presented April 10, 1940, at the 99th meeting of The American Chemical Society.

48. Green, M. and Greene, H., Eds. 1984. The Role of the Gastrointestinal Tract in Nutrient Delivery. Academic Press. Orlando.

49. Gruskin, B. 1940. Chlorophyll — its therapeutic place in acute and suppurative disease. American Journal of Surgery 49:49-55.

50. Guthrie, H. 1983. Introductory Nutrition (5th edition). C.V. Mosby Company. St. Louis.

51. Guyton, A. 1986. Textbook of Medical Physiology (7th Edition). W. B. Saunders Company, Philadelphia.

52. Hamilton, E., Whitney, E., and Sizer, F. 1988. Nutrition: Concepts and Controversies (4th Edition). West Publishing Co. St. Paul, Minn.

53. Hamilton, J. 1989. The National Research Council on diet and chronic disease. Physician's Weekly 6:14.

54. Hammel-Dupont, C. and Bessman, S. 1970. The stimulation of hemoglobin synthesis by porphyrins. Biochemical Medicine 4:55-60.

55. Hagiwara, Y. 1985. Green Barley Essence. Keats Publishing, New Canaan, CT.

56. Hansen, R., Scott, H. Larson, B. Nelson, T. and Krichevsky, P. 1953. Growth stimulation and growth inhibition of chicks fed forage and forage juice concentrate. Journal of Nutrition 49:453-464.

57. Howell, E. 1980. Food Enzymes for Health and Longevity. Omangod Press, Woodstock Valley, CT.

58. Hughes, J. and Latner, A. 1936. Chlorophyll and haemoglobin regeneration after haemorrhage. Journal of Physiology 86:388-395.

59. Illingsworth, C. 1939. Haemorrhage in jaundice. The Lancet 236:1031-1035.

60. Ingelfinger, F. 1968. For want of an enzyme. Nutrition Today 3:2-10.

61. Kahn, E.J. 1985. The Staffs of Life. Little, Brown & Co. Boston.

62. Kimm, S., Tschai, B., and Park, S. 1982. Antimutagenic activity of chlorophyll to direct and indirect-acting mutagens and its contents in the vegetables. Korean Journal of Biochemistry 14:1-7.

63. Kirschner, H. 1960. Nature's Healing Grasses. H. C. White Publications. Riverside, CA.

64. Kohler, G. 1953. The unidentified vitamins of grass and alfalfa. Feedstuffs, August 8, 1953.

65. Kohler, G. 1944. The effect of stages of growth on the chemistry of the grasses. The Journal of Biological Chemistry 152:215-223.

66. Kohler, G. 1939. Relation of pyrrole-containing pigments to hemoglobin synthesis. Journal of Biological Chemistry. 128:501-509.

67. Kohler, G., Elvehjem, C. and Hart, E. 1936. Growth stimulating properties of grass juice. Science. May 8, 1936, p.445.

68. Kohler, G. and Knuckles, B. 1977. Edible protein from leaves. Food Technology. May,1977.

69. Kohler, G., Randle, S. and Wagner, J. 1939. The Grass Juice Factor. Journal of Biological Chemistry. 128:lv.

70. Koo, L., 1988. Dietary habits and lung cancer risk among Chinese females in Hong Kong who never smoked. Nutrition and Cancer 11:155-72.

71. Kotzsch, R. E. 1988. The great green foods debate. East West Journal. July, 1988. 68-74.

72. Kubota, K. and Matsuoka, Y. 1984. Effect of chronic administration of green barley juice on growth rate, serum cholesterol level and internal organs of mice. Univ. of Tokyo. (no journal citation)

73. Kubota, K. and Matsuoka, Y. 1983. Isolation of potent anti-inflammatory protein from barley leaves. Japanese Journal of Inflammation 3(4).

74. Kubota, K. and Sunagane 1984. Studies on the effects of green barley juice on the endurance and motor activity in mice. Univ. of Tokyo. (no journal citation)

75. Kulvinskas, V. 1976. Survival Into the Twenty-First Century. Omangod Press. Wethersfield, CT.

76. Kune, G. and Kune, S. 1987. The nutritional causes of colorectal cancer: An introduction to the Melbourne Study. Nutrition and Cancer 9:1-4.

77. La Vecchia, C., Decarli, A., Negri, E., Parazzani, F., Gentile, A., Cecchetti, G., Fasoli, M., and Franceschi, S. 1987. Dietary factors and the risk of epithelial ovarian cancer. Journal of the National Cancer Institute 79:663-9.

78. La Vecchia, C., Negri, E., Decarli, A., Davanzo, B., and Franceschi, S. 1987. A case-control study of diet and gastric cancer in Northern Italy. International Journal of Cancer 40(4):484-9.

79. Lai, C. 1978. Chlorophyll: The active factor in wheat sprout extract inhibiting the metabolic activation of carcinogens in vitro. Nutritional Cancer 1:19-21.

80. Lai, C., Butler, M., and Matney, T. 1980. Antimutagenic activities of common vegetables and their chlorophyll content. Mutation Research 77:245-250.

81. Lai, C., Dabney, B., and Shaw, C. 1978. Inhibition of in vitro metabolic activation of carcinogens of wheat sprout extracts. Nutrition and Cancer 1:27-30.

82. Lakhanpal, R., Davis, J., Typpo, J., and Briggs, G. 1966. Evidence for an unidentified growth factor from alfalfa and other plant sources for young guinea pigs. Journal of Nutrition 89:341-346.

83. Langer, R. 1972. How Grasses Grow. Clowes & Sons.

84. Lappe, F. 1971. Diet for a Small Planet. Friends of the Earth/Ballentine Books. New York

85. Levy, L., Weintraub, D., and Fox, F. 1936. The food value of some common edible leaves. South African Medical Journal.10:699-707.

86. Locniskar, Mary. 1988. Nutrition and Health Symposium: The University of Texas at Austin, April 1988, Summary Report. Nutrition Today. Sept/Oct 1988:31-37.

87. McAuliffe, K. Gilbert, D. Kisttner, W., and Weir, D. 1987. How safe is your food? U.S. News and World Report Nov. 16, 1987.

88. McDougall, J.A. 1985. McDougall's Medicine: A Challenging Second Opinion New Century Publishers, Inc. New Jersey.

89. Milgrom, L. 1985. Chlorophyll is thicker than water. New Scientist. March 21, 1985, p.12.

90. Miller, J., Jackson, D. and Collier, C. 1960. The inhibition of Russell's viper venom by the water-soluble derivatives of sodium-copper chlorophyllin. American Journal of Surgery 99:48-49.

91. Miller, J., Jackson, D. and Collier, C. 1958. The inhibition of clotting by chlorophyllin. American Journal of Surgery 95:967-969.

92. Milton, K. and Demment, M. 1988. Digestion and passage kinetics of chimpanzees fed high and low fiber diets and comparison with human data. The Journal of Nutrition 118:1082-1088.

93. Muto, T. 1977. Therapeutic experiment of Bakuryokuso for the treatment of skin diseases in the main. "Muto Dermatologic Hospital". Vol. 26, #5.

94. Nagai, H. Nishiyori, T. Daikoku, M. and Koda, A. 1983. Immunopharmacological studies of sodium copper chlorophyllin. Japanese Journal of Pharmacology 33:819-28.

95. Naisbitt, J. 1988. The healing power of food. New Age September/ October, 1988. 25.

96. New Scientist, April 12, 1984. Monitor: Why a Lost Soldier Should Eat Grass.

97. Niwa, Y. and Miyachi, Y. 1986. Antioxidant action of natural health products and Chinese herbs. Inflammation 10:79-91.

98. Nutrition Search, Inc. 1984. Nutrition Almanac. McGraw-Hill. New York.

99. Offenkrantz, W. 1950. Water-soluble chlorophyll in the treatment of peptic ulcers of long duration. Review of Gastroenterology 17:359-367.

100. Ohno, Y., Yoshida, O., Oishi, K., Okada, K., Yamabe, H. Schroeder, F. 1988. Dietary beta-carotene and cancer of the prostate: a case-control study in Kyoto. Cancer Research 48(5):1331-6.

101. Ohtake, H., Nonaka, S., Sawada,Y., Hagiwara, Y., Hagiwara, H.,and Kubota, K. 1985. Studies on the constituents of green juice from young barley leaves. Effect on dietarily induced hypercholesterolemia in rats. Journal of the Pharmaceutical Society of Japan 105:1052-71.

102. Ohtake, H., Yuasa, H., Komura, C. Miyauchi, T., Hagiwara, Y., Kubota, K. 1985. Studies on the constituents of green juice from young barley leaves. Antiulcer activity of fractions from barley juice. Journal of the Pharmaceutical Society of Japan 105:1046-51.

103. Ong, T., Whong, W. Stewart, J., and Brockman, H. 1989. Comparative antimutagenicity of 5 compounds against 5 mutagenic complex mixtures in Salmonella typhimurium strain TA98. Mutation Research 222:19-25.

104. Ong, T., Whong, W., Stewart, J. and Brockman, H. 1986. Chlorophyllin: a potent antimutagen against environmental and dietary complex mixtures. Mutation Research 173:111-15.

105. Patek, A. 1936. Chlorophyll and regeneration of the blood. Archives of Internal Medicine 57:73-84.

106. Patek, A. and Minot, G. 1934. The effect of bile pigment in cases of chronic hypochromic anemia. American Journal of Medical Sciences 188:206-215.

107. Peoples, M., Frith, G., and Dalling, M. 1979. Proteolytic enzymes in green wheat leaves IV. Degradation of ribulose 1,5-biphosphate carboxylase by acid proteinases isolated on DEAE-cellulose. Plant and Cell Physiology 20:253-258.

108. Pike, A. (quoting Y. Hagiwara) 1982. Barley, a green revolution. Let's Live. March,1982.

109. Pirie, N. 1969. The present position of research on the use of leaf protein as a human food. Plant Foods and Human Nutrition 1:237-246.

110. Pisani, P., Berrino, F., Macaluso, M., Pastorino, U., Crosignani, and Baldasseroni, A. 1986. Carrots, green vegetables and lung cancer: A case-control study. International Journal of Epidemiology 15:463-468.

111. Rafsky, H. and Krieger, C. 1948. The treatment of intestinal diseases with solutions of water-soluble chlorophyll. Review of Gastroenterology 15:549-553.

112. Raj, A. and Katz, M. 1985. Beta-carotene as an inhibitor of benzo(a)pyrene and mitomycin C induced chromosomal breaks in the bone marrow of mice. Canadian Journal of Genetics and Cytology 27:598-602.

113. Randle, S. Sober, H. and Kohler, G. 1940. The distribution of the grass juice factor in plant and animal materials. Journal of Nutrition 20:459-466.

114. Ravdin, L. 1939. Problems of long standing gallstone disease. Kansas City Medical Journal. Feb, 1939.

115. Rhoads, J. 1939. The relation of vitamin K to the hemorrhagic tendency in obstructive jaundice with a report on cerophyll as a source of vitamin K. Surgery 5:794-808.

116. Robinson, A. 1979. Diet and Cancer. in: Barron's Mailbag. Barron's. September 3,1979.p.7.

117. Rosen, E. 1987. Interview: Viktoras Kulvinskas. Whole Life September/October 1987. 37.

118. Roshevits, R. 1937. Grasses—An Introduction to the Study of Fodder and Cereal Grasses. Translated from the original Russian for the Smithsonian Institute and the National Science Foundation, 1980.

119. Rothemund, P., McNary, R., and Inman, O. 1934. Occurrence of decomposition products of chlorophyll.II. Decomposition products of chlorophyll in the stomach walls of herbivorous animals. Journal of the American Chemical Society 56:2400-2403.

120. Sack, P., and Barnard, R. 1955. Studies on the hemagglutinating and inflammation properties of exudate from nonhealing wounds and their inhibition by chlorophyll derivatives. New York State Journal of Medicine. October 15, 1955, p.2952-2956.

121. Saunders, C. 1926. The nutritional value of chlorophyll as related to hemoglobin formation. Proceedings of the Society for Experimental Biology and Medicine (3172)p.788-789.

122. Schnabel, C. 1940. We're harvesting our crops too late! Magazine Digest. November, 1940.

123. Schnabel, C. 1935. The biologic value of high protein cereal grasses. Paper presented to the biologic section of the American Chemical Society in New York, April 22, 1935.

124. Schultz, D. 1979. Sprouts vs Cancer? Checkup on Medicine in: Science News. May,1979, p.78.

125. Scott, E. and Delor, C. 1933. Nutritional anemia. Ohio State Medical Journal 29:165-169.

126. Scott, M. 1986. Nutrition of Humans and Selected Animal Species. John Wiley and Sons. New York.

127. Seely, S., Freed, D., Silverstone, G., Rippere, V. Diet Related Diseases, The Modern Epidemic. Croom Helm. London & Sydney. 1985.

128. Siegel, L. 1960. The control of ileostomy and colostomy odors. Gastroenterology 38:634-6.

129. Sinclair, H. 1979. The human nutritional advantages of plant foods over animal foods. Qualitas Planitas—Plant Foods in Human Nutrition 29:7-18.

130. Singleton, J. 1940. A measure in the treatment of menorrhagia. Kansas City Medical Journal. March, 1940.

131. Smith, L. 1955. The present status of topical chlorophyll therapy. The NY State Journal of Medicine. July 15, 1955, p. 2041-2049.

132. Smith, L. 1944. Chlorophyll: an experimental study of its water-soluble derivatives. Remarks on the history, chemistry, toxicity and anti-bacterial properties of water soluble chlorophyll derivatives as therapeutic agents. American Journal of the Medical Sciences 207:647-654.

133. Spector, H. and Calloway, D. 1959. Reduction of x-radiation mortality by cabbage and broccoli. Proceedings of the Society for Experimental Biology and Medicine 100:405-407.

134. Spitzer, R. and Phillips, P. 1946. Reproduction and lactation studies with rats fed natural rations. Journal of Nutrition 32:631-639.

135. Subar, A., Block, G., James, L. 1989. Folate intake and food sources in the U.S. population. American Journal of Clinical Nutrition 50:508-16.

136. Surgeon General's Report on Nutrition and Health, Summary and Recommendations. Nutrition Today. Sept,1988.

137. Sussman, R., 1987. Morpho-physiological analysis of diets: species-specific dietary patterns in primates and human dietary adaptations in: The Evolution of Human Behavior: Primate Models. W. Kinzey, Ed. State University of New York Press. Albany.

138. Tangley, L. 1987. Regulating pesticides in foods. Bioscience 37:452-456.

139. Verreault, R., Chu, J., Mandelson, M. and Shy, K. 1989. A case-control study of diet and invasive cervical cancer. International Journal of Cancer 43(6):1050-4.

140. von Wendt, G. 1935. A recently discovered nutritive factor in milk. Reviewed in Kohler (1953).

141. Wagner, J. 1989. Agricide, an interview with Dr. Michael Fox. Clarion Call 1(4):19.

142. Walker, A., Walker, B., and Wadvalla, M. 1975. An attempt to measure the availability of calcium in edible leaves commonly consumed by South African Negroes. Ecology of Food and Nutrition 4:125-30.

143. Watson, R. Ed. 1984. Nutrition, Disease Resistance, and Immune Function. Marcel Dekker. New York.

144. Whong, W., Stewart, J., Brockman, H. and Ong, T. 1988. Comparative antimutagenicity of chlorophyllin and five other agents against aflatoxin B1 induced reversion in salmonella typhimurium strain TA98. Teratogenesis, Carcinogenesis, and Mutagenesis 8:215-24.

145. Wigmore, A. 1985. The Wheatgrass Book. Avery Publishing Group. Wayne, NJ.

146. Wille, C., 1987. Death on Your Dinner Table. NAS Briefings, Audubon 89:130.

147. Wills, E. 1985. Biochemical Basis of Medicine. John Wright & Sons, Bristol.

148. Wilson, C. 1961. Grass and People. University of Florida Press. Gainesville.

149. Wilson, J. and Wilson, A. 1967. Grassland. Wide Skies Press. Polk, NE.

150. Woolley, D.and Krampitz, L. 1943. Production of a scurvy-like condition by feeding of a compound structurally related to ascorbic acid. Journal of Experimental Medicine 78:333.

151. Young, R. and Beregi, J. 1980. Use of chlorophyllin in the care of geriatric patients. Journal of the American Geriatrics Society 28:46-47.

152. Ziegler, R., Mason, T., Stemhagen, A., Hoover, R., Schoenberg, J., Gridley, G., Virgo, P., and Fraumeni, J. 1986. Carotenoid intake, vegetables, and the risk of lung cancer among white men in New Jersey. American Journal of Epidemiology 123:1080-1093.

153. Laboratory Analyses, September 6, 1989. Nutrition International, East Brunswick, NJ.

Appendix A

Cereal Grass and Allergies

Those who are allergic to wheat and other grain products are almost never allergic to the green cereal grasses. Allergies to wheat, barley and rye products are usually reactions to **gluten**, the tenacious elastic protein substance that gives cohesiveness to bread dough. The cereal grasses do not contain gluten. Their chemical profiles are like those of other leafy green vegetables, and unlike those of grains, or mature cereal seeds. A few people who are allergic to dark green vegetables or to a variety of grasses are occasionally also allergic to the cereal grasses.

Allergy-prone individuals need to take special care to eat a well balanced and nutritionally adequate diet to sustain their general good health, and particularly their immune systems. Allergies are **hyper**-immune reactions; when the immune system cannot tolerate an offending substance (the allergen), it mounts a defense against things which are harmless to most of us. This situation puts stress on the allergic person's immune system.

Little research has been done on the best ways for allergic people to counter this stress nutritionally, but the nutrients generally thought to support and enhance the immune system include vitamin C, beta-carotene and vitamin A, protein, iron, calcium, and the B complex vitamins. Fiber might also be helpful by diluting and enhancing the elimination of the offending substance in the digestive tract. Chlorophyll, with its general detoxifying properties, could also be beneficial in this regard. A chlorophyll derivative has been shown to inhibit allergy reactions (Types I, II, and III) in laboratory rats.[94]

There is sufficient reason, then, to believe that increasing one's intake of dark green vegetables may provide positive benefits for one's immunological health. Those with wheat or barley allergies can generally consume wheat grass and barley grass with no allergic reaction, and provide their immune systems with the benefits of the wide range of nutrients concentrated in these simple green foods.

Appendix B

Nutrient Values of Commonly Consumed Green Food Supplements

	Dehydrated Wheat Grass whole leaf (U.S.A.)	Dehydrated Barley Leaf juice extract (Japan)	Dehydrated Alfalfa whole leaf (U.S.A.)	Dehydrated Spirulina (Mexico)
Chlorophyll (mg./100g.)	543	186	168	528
Beta-Carotene (IU/100g.)	23,136	4,795	4,524	22,109
Iron (mg./100g.)	33.7	4.68	75.4	44.88
Crude Fiber (%)	16.51	1.36	25.0	1.79
Protein (%)	22.13	19.85	17.5	53.88
Fat (%)	6.49	12.76	*	6.08

*No data available

Sources: References 64 and 153.

INDEX